THE HORMONAL PAUSES

The Menopause Brain Reset, Relief, Support, Diet Plan, Weight Loss and Understanding the Transformations in Your Body.

BY SUMMER HALL

COPYRIGHT

DISCLAIMER

The information provided in this book is intended for general informational purposes only and is not a substitute for professional advice or treatment. While the author has made every effort to ensure the accuracy and completeness of the information presented, readers are encouraged to consult with qualified healthcare professionals, educators, or mental health practitioners for personalized advice and guidance tailored to their specific needs and circumstances.

The author and publisher disclaim any liability or responsibility for any loss, injury, or damage incurred as a result of the use or reliance on the information provided in this book. The reader assumes full responsibility for their own actions and decisions based on the information presented herein.

This book may contain references to third-party websites, resources, or products for informational purposes. The inclusion of such references does not imply endorsement or recommendation by the author or publisher. Readers are encouraged to independently verify the accuracy and suitability of any information or resource mentioned in this book.

By reading this book, the reader acknowledges and agrees to the terms of this disclaimer.

Letter To the Reader

I appreciate you taking the time to read this.

THE HORMONAL PAUSES aims to provide a thorough manual for overcoming menopause with resilience and confidence by balancing knowledge, emotional support, and self-care strategies.

This book seeks to demystify menopause through lucid, empirically supported explanations of the biological processes at each stage—perimenopause, menopause, and post menopause.

THE HORMONAL PAUSES aims to equip women to embrace each stage of menopause with a mentality that values self-acceptance, personal development, and holistic well-being, in addition to providing them with knowledge. It exposes those menopausal symptoms that people don't talk about.

By taking this approach, the book hopes to change menopause from a terrifying topic to one that empowers readers.

It's not all in your head, and you're not alone.

Introduction

The significance of menopause as a natural phase in a woman's life

Menopause is a natural stage that signifies the end of a woman's reproductive years, it's a significant life transition that goes well beyond a medical milestone. Menopause should not be seen as an end, but rather as a substantial shift that leads to new phases of well-being, self-acceptance, and personal development.

Menopause marks the start of a stage frequently characterized by more self-awareness and clarity. Many women report feeling more focused and connected to their own beliefs and objectives after being released from the hormonal swings linked to conception.

Many women experience respite from menstrual cycle problems, such as monthly cramps, PMS, or having to deal with birth control issues, after their periods are over. Given that women often place a higher value on physical attributes like bone health, cardiovascular fitness, and mental clarity, this physical change permits more flexibility and an emphasis on whole-body health. Therefore, menopause is not about losing health but refocusing on lifespan and sustained self-care.

Although many civilizations now view menopause as a period of strength and liberation, historically it was linked to ageing and loss.

Menopause can be an emotional period of introspection and identity transformation.

Menopause is genuinely a transition—a springboard to a stage of life characterized by self-reliance, self-acceptance, and a revitalized sense of purpose. Women may cultivate resilience, wisdom, and energy in their post-menopausal years by seeing this transition as a significant life event rather than an "end." This will help them adopt a healthier, more holistic perspective on ageing and well-being.

The Three Stages (perimenopause, menopause, and post menopause)

Perimenopause, menopause, and post menopause are the three separate stages of menopause, each of which has its own set of symptoms and hormonal changes. Comprehending these phases can enable women to foresee changes, make knowledgeable decisions regarding their health, and confidently embrace each phase.

1. Perimenopause: The Phase of Transition

The transitional period before menopause is known as perimenopause, and it usually starts in a woman's 40s, though it can start younger. Estrogen and progesterone levels begin to change during this phase, which can result in mood swings, hot flashes, irregular menstruation periods, and disturbed sleep, understanding that perimenopause marks the start of hormonal shifts aids women in preparing for impending changes. When individuals recognize this stage, they can start making lifestyle changes, look for ways to control their symptoms and start talking to medical professionals about measures like diet, exercise, and perhaps even low-dose hormone therapy.

2. Menopause: The Turning Point

A woman enters menopause when she has not had a menstrual period for 12 months in a row, usually around age 51. The reproductive years are over because the ovaries have drastically decreased their hormone output. Night sweats, hot flushes, and changes in bone density and libido are typical symptoms.

3. Post menopause- The New Chapter After Menopause

After menopause, a woman has post menopause, which lasts the remainder of her life. Some symptoms, such as hot flashes, may persist, although they usually subside with time as hormone levels settle at lower levels. However, because of decreased estrogen levels, this period increases the risk of diseases like osteoporosis and heart disease. Knowing the possible health hazards and advantages of post menopause, women can make informed choices about diet, exercise and medical treatments.

Knowledge Is Power

Understanding these phases enables women to make plans, seek help, and modify their lifestyles to improve their mental and physical well-being. You may turn menopause into a period of empowerment and rejuvenation by seeing each stage as a natural evolution rather than a decline.

Table of Contents

PART ONE

1. Understanding Hormonal Pauses

The Science of Menopause

The roles of key hormones like estrogen, progesterone, and testosterone in a woman's body.

Significant hormonal changes, especially in the levels of estrogen, progesterone, and testosterone, are characteristic of the complicated biological transition known as menopause. Each of these hormones is essential in controlling a variety of body processes; a fall in them causes many of the physical and mental symptoms linked with menopause.

1. The Main Regulator: Estrogen

Function in the Body: One of the key female sex hormones, estrogen, is in charge of the development and maintenance of breast and reproductive tissues and the regulation of the monthly cycle. It affects bone density, heart health, skin elasticity, and even mood and cognition in addition to reproductive functions.

During perimenopause, estrogen levels steadily drop as women get closer to menopause, resulting in swings that induce symptoms including hot flashes, night sweats, and mood swings.

Since estrogen preserves bone density and healthy blood arteries, lower estrogen levels are also associated with a higher risk of osteoporosis and heart disease after menopause.

Effects on the Brain: Estrogen regulates neurotransmitters, which impact mood and cognitive abilities. Since estrogen has been shown to interact with serotonin, a neurotransmitter involved in mood stability, lower levels can cause symptoms including mood swings, forgetfulness, and brain fog.

2. Progesterone: The Regulator

Function in the Body: Progesterone balances the effects of estrogen on the body, preparing the uterus for pregnancy, and controlling the menstrual cycle. It has a soothing impact on the brain, which may help to lower anxiety and encourage sound sleep.

Changes During Menopause: Progesterone levels frequently start to drop in perimenopause, sometimes more abruptly than estrogen. Disturbances in mood, sleep, and menstrual cycles can all be caused by this imbalance. Estrogen dominance, which can result from a relative decrease in progesterone relative to estrogen, can also induce perimenopausal symptoms such as bloating, breast pain, and irritability.

Effect on Mood and Sleep: Because progesterone calms the brain, decreased levels can cause anxiety and sleep problems, which are typical complaints among menopausal women. The decline of this hormone is frequently linked to poor sleep and heightened susceptibility to stress throughout menopause.

3. Testosterone: The Silent Helper

Function in the Body: Although testosterone is frequently associated with men, it also plays a significant role in the health of women. It enhances libido, energy levels, bone strength, and muscular mass. Typically, women have lower testosterone levels compared to males, but they contribute to preserving a feeling of health and vigor.

Changes During Menopause: As people age, testosterone levels in both men and women steadily decrease, but in postmenopausal women, this loss is more noticeable. Reduced libido, muscular mass, and energy are all linked to lower testosterone levels. Some women might consider using testosterone treatment as part of their menopausal management strategy, although there are conflicting views regarding the safety and effectiveness of this current study issue.

Impact on Sexual Health: Since testosterone sustains sexual desire, postmenopausal women's libido and sexual pleasure may be affected by its decline. Using therapy or changing one's lifestyle to address these changes can help many women deal with these elements of menopause health effectively.

The Interplay of Hormones

Numerous physical and mental elements of menopause are largely dependent on the complex balance of estrogen, progesterone, and testosterone. Knowing the functions of these hormones as they diminish might enable women to pursue specific therapies and lifestyle modifications to promote their health both during and beyond menopause. Supplements, lifestyle modifications, and hormone replacement therapy (HRT) can all be useful strategies for symptom management; nevertheless, a healthcare professional should always be consulted for individualized treatment.

Women may take proactive measures to preserve well-being, control symptoms, and welcome menopause as a time of transition and development by learning more about these hormonal shifts.

How these hormones impact various systems in the body.

Numerous bodily systems depend on the hormones testosterone, progesterone, and estrogen; these hormone levels have a major effect on the brain, bones, heart, and other systems as they fluctuate and eventually fall throughout menopause, which contributes to the mental and physical changes that occur during this phase.

1. The brain

Estrogen: Estrogen has a profound impact on the brain. It aids in regulating neurotransmitters (serotonin and Dopamine) that affect mood and emotional stability; due to the effects of these brain chemicals, mood swings, anxiety, and even depression can result from changing estrogen levels during perimenopause. Estrogen also facilitates the metabolism of brain energy by encouraging the intake of glucose, which is critical for mental clarity and cognitive performance. Therefore, symptoms such as brain fog, memory lapses and difficulty concentrating may increase by declining estrogen levels throughout menopause.

Progesterone: Often known as the "calming hormone," progesterone calms the brain. Gamma-aminobutyric acid (GABA), a neurotransmitter that encourages relaxation and lowers anxiety, is activated more when present. Progesterone reduction during perimenopause and menopause may increase tension, anxiety, and sleep disruptions.

Testosterone: This hormone also affects motivation, mood, and mental energy, all aspects of cognitive wellness. Reduced attention and mental acuity may result from its steady reduction throughout menopause. Although testosterone levels are lower in women than in males, this hormone promotes emotions of vitality and can affect mental health when it decreases.

2. Bones

Estrogen: The maintenance of bone density depends on estrogen. By regulating the activity of osteoclasts, (cells that break down bone), it aids in regulating bone remodeling and osteoblasts (bone-building cells). Bone resorption frequently surpasses bone creation as estrogen levels fall after menopause, resulting in bone loss and an elevated risk of osteoporosis. This puts postmenopausal women at heightened risk for fractures, particularly in the wrists, hips, and spine. Weight-bearing activities, calcium, vitamin D, and occasionally prescription drugs are advised to support bone health following menopause.

Progesterone: Although indirectly, progesterone also affects bone health. Its presence enhances the effects of estrogen by promoting the production of new bone. Therefore, in postmenopausal women, a decrease in progesterone may worsen the loss of bone density.

Testosterone: Promotes bone density, even though it is mostly linked to muscle mass. Low testosterone levels can cause weaker bones, increasing the dangers of osteoporosis when estrogen and progesterone levels are also low.

This is why certain postmenopausal therapies take into account testosterone supplements, even if research on their safety and effectiveness is still ongoing.

3. Heart and Cardiovascular System

Estrogen: The cardiovascular system is protected by estrogen. By encouraging vasodilation, (relaxing blood vessels and increasing blood flow), it maintains normal blood vessel function. By increasing HDL (High-Density Lipoprotein), or the "good" cholesterol, and decreasing LDL (Low-Density Lipoprotein), or the "bad" cholesterol, estrogen also helps maintain healthy cholesterol levels. Women are more susceptible to heart disease when their estrogen levels drop after menopause because these preventative benefits are lessened.

Progesterone: Although it has a less noticeable direct effect on the cardiovascular system, progesterone may assist in lowering blood pressure by balancing fluid levels in conjunction with estrogen. Its decrease after menopause could obliquely cause heart-related symptoms, especially when combined with other cardiovascular changes associated with ageing.

Testosterone: This hormone also contributes to heart health. Low levels can result in decreased cardiac muscle strength and endurance. While research on testosterone's effects on women's cardiovascular health is ongoing, some data points to its potential to improve heart function and preserve blood vessel flexibility.

4. Additional Systems Affected by Hormonal Shifts

Muscles and Skin: Muscle mass maintenance and skin elasticity depend on testosterone and estrogen. When these hormone levels fall, women may suffer from decreased muscular mass, muscle weakness, and skin changes including thinning, wrinkles, and dryness. Strength training and skincare routines are therefore frequently advised for women undergoing menopause to assist in lessening these impacts.

Distribution of Fat and Metabolism: Estrogen affects the body's fat storage. As estrogen levels fall, the distribution of fat frequently moves from the thighs and hips to the belly, raising the risk of visceral fat, which is associated with an increased risk of cardiovascular disease. A decrease in testosterone can lead to changes in body composition and decreased energy, which makes weight control more difficult because testosterone also affects metabolism and energy levels.

In conclusion,

Estrogen, progesterone, and testosterone interact to influence several bodily systems, and many of the physical and mental symptoms that women have can be explained by their drop after menopause. Comprehending these effects enables women to take charge of their health through dietary adjustments, lifestyle modifications, and medical advice.

Debunking Myths about Menopause

Despite being a normal aspect of life, menopause is surrounded by a lot of myths and misconceptions that might distort women's expectations or generate needless anxiety. Accurate information is crucial to debunk these beliefs and enable women to navigate this stage.

Myth 1: Menopause Indicates You Are "Old"

Fact: Menopause is only a hormonal shift that signifies the end of the reproductive years. It usually happens at about age 51. However, it can come earlier or later. It is not synonymous with ageing in terms of mental or physical deterioration. Many women use this time to concentrate on their careers, personal development, or other goals in life. Menopause is a time of life that may be full of life and independence from the monthly menstrual cycle.

Myth 2: Menopause Is the Same for Every Woman

Fact: Every woman has a different menopausal experience. Some people may go through menopause with few symptoms, while others may have severe symptoms like mood swings, hot flashes, and night sweats. Each woman's experience of menopause is unique and influenced by several factors, including lifestyle, genetics, and general health. Knowing this uniqueness enables women to avoid pointless comparisons and create individualized treatment plans.

Myth 3: Hormone Treatment Is Risky

Fact: Hormone therapy, especially estrogen therapy, was formerly commonly used to treat menopausal symptoms until concerns arose over potential links to cancer and heart disease. However, further studies have demonstrated that when well controlled, HT can be safe and helpful, particularly for women who are in the early stages of menopause (under 60 or within ten years of the commencement of menopause). The

The decision to take HT is personal and should be discussed with a healthcare professional to balance the dangers and benefits.

Myth 4: Your Sexual Life Ends with Menopause

Fact: Although menopause might alter libido and sexual health, it does not mean that closeness or sexual pleasure is over. Although lubricants, vaginal estrogen, and other treatments are available, lower estrogen levels can induce vaginal dryness, which can make intercourse painful. Some women also report feeling more sexually interested again because of things like not having to worry about getting pregnant. By keeping lines of communication open with partners and investigating various possibilities for comfort and enjoyment, you can have an enjoyable sex life.

Myth 5: Menopause Symptoms Are Unavoidable

Fact: Menopausal symptoms can be managed using lifestyle changes, a healthy diet, frequent exercise, and stress reduction; these are the cornerstones of symptom treatment. HT and cognitive behavioral therapy, as well as medications and herbal supplements, can be used for symptoms like mood swings, sleep difficulties, and hot flashes. Numerous resources, support groups, and medical specialists in menopausal care are available.

Myth 6: Severe Mental Decline Occurs During Menopause

Fact: Although hormone fluctuations might result in short-term cognitive abnormalities like forgetfulness or brain fog, they are often transient. Menopause does not cause substantial or irreversible mental impairment, according to studies, and when hormonal fluctuations have subsided, cognitive performance frequently returns to normal. Activities that promote brain health and help control cognitive symptoms after menopause include mental exercise, getting enough sleep, and physical activity.

Myth7: Menopause Is Equivalent to Weight Gain

Fact: Menopause does not directly cause weight gain, even if hormonal changes might affect metabolism and alter weight distribution. Weight gain at this period is frequently brought on by age, decreased muscle mass, and lifestyle choices. Women can efficiently maintain their weight during and after menopause by putting an emphasis on strength training, a healthy diet, and frequent exercise.

Conclusion: Why Accurate Information Matters

Women who have access to accurate information are better able to view menopause as a natural stage with controllable symptoms rather than a deterioration. Knowledgeable women are better able to establish supportive practices, make educated health decisions, and navigate this shift with confidence. By dispelling these beliefs, society may change its perspective on menopause to one that values development, fortitude, and wisdom, eventually assisting women in accepting this change healthily.

2: Perimenopause

Early Signs and Symptoms, and Body Changes

The time before menopause, when a woman's body starts to experience hormonal changes, is known as perimenopause. Though the exact time varies from person to person, this phase usually begins in a woman's late 30s to early 40s. With an average duration of four years, perimenopause can last anywhere from a few months to almost ten years. When a woman has not had her period for 12 months in a row, perimenopause ends and menopause begins.

What Triggers Perimenopause?

Perimenopause is triggered by changes in the production of reproductive hormones, primarily estrogen and progesterone, as the ovaries begin to age and gradually lose efficiency. Contrary to menopause, which is a permanent stop in the synthesis of hormones, perimenopause is characterized by fluctuating levels of estrogen and progesterone.

In the latter phases of perimenopause, these hormonal changes intensify as estrogen levels gradually but erratically drop.

Hormonal Changes During Perimenopause

Estrogen: Unpredictable fluctuations in estrogen levels lead to irregular menstrual periods. Many typical perimenopausal symptoms, including mood swings, hot flashes, and breast pain, are caused by sudden reductions in estrogen levels, after high levels.

Progesterone: Periods become irregular and may be heavier or lighter than usual because of decreased progesterone production brought on by fewer ovulations.

Testosterone: Despite the slower rate of reduction, testosterone does have a role in changes in muscle mass, libido, and energy levels throughout this period.

Signs of the Perimenopause

Although every woman's perimenopausal experience is unique, typical symptoms include:

Irregular Periods: As ovulation becomes irregular, periods may become heavier, lighter, longer, or shorter. Some women may have periods that are closer together than usual or skip months.

Hot Flashes and Night Sweats: Hormonal changes can cause sudden sensations of heat, usually followed by redness and perspiration.

Mood Changes: Women may be more prone to mood swings, impatience, and occasionally sadness or anxiety.

These alterations are connected to variations in estrogen, which impacts mood-regulating neurotransmitters.

Sleep Disturbances: Night sweats and insomnia can cause sleep disturbances, which results in daytime exhaustion and diminished mental acuity.

Reduced Libido and Vaginal Dryness: Vaginal dryness brought on by low estrogen levels may make sexual activity uncomfortable. Libido changes are also common.

Age Range

A woman's perimenopause usually starts in her late 30s or early 40s. While "late perimenopause" is more prevalent around the end of the 40s, "early perimenopause," often referred to as "early perimenopause," can begin before that age. The time of perimenopause can be influenced by some factors like lifestyle, stress levels, genetics, and general health. Perimenopause can cause significant physical and mental changes for some women, while it is hardly evident for others.

Managing the Symptoms of Perimenopause

Despite being a normal stage, perimenopause symptoms can be managed by self-care techniques, medical assistance, and lifestyle changes:

Diet and Exercise: Bone and hormonal health can be improved by a well-balanced diet high in calcium, vitamin D, and phytoestrogens (such as soy products). Frequent exercise is beneficial, particularly strength training.

Stress Reduction: Yoga, meditation, and relaxation techniques can help reduce stress, which can make perimenopausal symptoms worse.

Hormonal and Non-Hormonal Treatments: Depending on the individual needs of each woman, low-dose birth control tablets or hormone therapy (HT) may be suggested to balance hormonal levels. Mood issues can also be effectively managed with non-hormonal therapies such as cognitive-behavioral therapy (CBT), herbal supplements, and antidepressants.

Why It's Important to Understand Perimenopause

Women who are aware of perimenopause are better able to accept this stage as a normal transition rather than an abrupt, inexplicable shift. Women may make proactive health decisions, seek help when necessary, and feel more in charge of their bodies and well-being at this period of life if they know what to expect.

Body Changes in Perimenopause

Hormonal changes during perimenopause affect how the body feels, looks, and functions, resulting in several physical changes. Weight distribution, skin texture, metabolism, and menstruation cycles are frequently affected by these changes, however, the effects vary from woman to woman.

1. Changes in Body Composition and Weight Distribution

Shift in Fat Storage: Estrogen levels fluctuate and decrease throughout the perimenopause. Estrogen affects fat distribution, stored around the hips and thighs. Lower levels of estrogen tend to cause a change in the distribution of fat, which increases belly fat. A higher risk of metabolic and cardiovascular illnesses is linked to this shift toward central or visceral fat.

Loss of Muscle Mass: Sarcopenia a progressive loss of muscle mass is brought on by decreased levels of estrogen and testosterone. As a result, muscle tone may decline, making it difficult to retain strength and simpler to acquire fat. To combat this loss and boost metabolism, resistance training and exercise are frequently advised.

2. Elasticity and Texture of the Skin

Dryness and Thinning: The creation of collagen, which is necessary for the suppleness and hydration of skin, is also influenced by estrogen. The skin becomes thinner, drier, and more prone to fine lines and wrinkles due to decreased collagen and skin hydration brought on by declining estrogen levels during perimenopause. Additionally, skin texture might change, becoming rougher and less elastic.

Sensitivity and Healing: Thinner skin may be more susceptible to irritations and heal more slowly. Many women change their skincare regimens to incorporate extra moisturizing, mild products and sun protection because this can make perimenopausal skin more prone to irritation, dryness, and bruising.

3. Changes in Metabolism

Reduced Metabolic Rate: Age-related metabolic slowdowns are normal, but perimenopausal hormone changes might worsen them. Lower levels of estrogen can make it easier to gain weight and more difficult to lose it because they influence insulin sensitivity and fat accumulation. Decreased testosterone also slows metabolism since muscle burns more calories than fat by nature. The body needs fewer calories to operate when the metabolism is slower, which increases the chance of weight gain if dietary habits aren't adjusted.

Blood Sugar Regulation and Insulin Sensitivity: Reduced estrogen levels may also result in less insulin sensitivity, which increases the likelihood of blood sugar swings. This metabolic alteration contributes to weight gain, especially around the belly, and can cause changes in appetite and increased desires, especially for sugary or high-carb meals.

4. Irregularities in Menstruation

Changes in Cycle Length and Flow: Menstrual cycles become less regular during perimenopause. The length of periods can change, as can their flow. This anomaly is brought on by varying amounts of progesterone and estrogen, which can lead to "anovulatory cycles," in which no egg is produced, or missed ovulations. Women may thus have lighter or noticeably heavier than normal periods, along with timing variations.

Hormonal Fluctuation Symptoms: Even if menstruation becomes uncommon, changes in estrogen and progesterone can result in symptoms that resemble those of PMS, such as bloating, mood swings, and breast soreness. Abrupt fluctuations in estrogen levels can also cause hot flashes and night sweats.

In summary,

Hormonal changes during the perimenopause cause notable physical changes. Menstrual periods become erratic, metabolism slows, skin is drier and less elastic, and weight is frequently transferred to the belly. Women aware of these changes should modify their self-care practices, such as exercise, skincare, and diet, to better handle and preserve their health.

Practical Advice for Managing Symptoms

Diet, stress management, and lifestyle changes are all components of a complete strategy for managing menopausal and perimenopausal symptoms. Here are some doable strategies to help women transition smoothly and improve their wellbeing:

1. Dietary Modifications

Eat more Phytoestrogens: Plant-based substances called phytoestrogens, which resemble estrogen in the body, are found in foods like soy, flaxseeds, and legumes. These meals may help lessen mood swings and hot flashes while offering natural hormonal support. However, especially for women with a history of estrogen-sensitive illnesses, phytoestrogen consumption should be balanced and addressed with a healthcare professional.

Increase Vitamin D and Calcium Consumption: Since bone density decreases more quickly when estrogen levels fall, it's critical to promote bone health by eating foods high in calcium, such as dairy, leafy greens, and fortified plant milk, and provide sufficient vitamin

D, which facilitates the absorption of calcium. Sunlight exposure, supplements, and meals like fatty fish and fortified goods can all provide vitamin D.

Use Omega-3s to Promote Heart Health: Incorporating omega-3 fatty acid sources (such as walnuts, chia seeds, and salmon) might improve heart health and perhaps lower inflammation, which enhances mental clarity and mood stability, this is because lower estrogen levels can raise cardiovascular risks.

Reduce Sugar and Caffeine Intake: Sugar and caffeine can worsen mood swings and hot flashes- raising adrenaline levels and causing rapid changes in blood sugar- lowering consumption and switching to healthier choices (like green tea) will help you keep your energy levels consistent.

2. Strategies for Stress Reduction

Regular mindfulness exercises, including deep breathing, meditation, or guided imagery, can help you become more emotionally resilient and less stressed. These exercises can lessen hot flashes and improve mood stability by relaxing the nervous system. Even just 5-10 minutes a day is beneficial for stress management and mental clarity.

Frequent Physical Activity: Exercise, especially strength training and aerobic activities, has been shown to reduce stress and improve general health. It can regulate weight, lower the risk of osteoporosis by strengthening bones and muscles, and elevate mood by generating endorphins. Moreover, mild workouts like yoga or Pilates can promote flexibility, ease stress, and promote relaxation.

Engage in Social Support and Connection: Connecting with loved ones, friends, or support organizations can comfort and give a chance to discuss menopausal experiences. Having a network of people who support you might help you feel less alone and encourage you during this change.

3. Lifestyle Changes

Sleep Hygiene for Better Sleep: Establishing a peaceful nighttime routine is crucial since perimenopause frequently causes sleep disturbances. Keep your bedroom cold, maintain a regular sleep schedule, and steer clear of screens and heavy meals just before bed. Additionally, reading or listening to relaxing music before bed might assist in enhancing the quality of your sleep.

Use Cooling Techniques for Hot Flashes: Wear layers of clothes that you can take off as required and keep cool water close at hand to help cool down. Some women find that natural cooling methods, such as applying a cold cloth on the forehead or using fans, can help reduce the intensity of hot flashes when they arise.

Limit Alcohol Consumption: Alcohol can exacerbate hot flashes, interfere with sleep, and cause mood changes. For individuals who are susceptible to its effects, cutting back on alcohol or consuming non-alcoholic alternatives might help regulate mood and enhance sleep.

A healthy diet, stress reduction techniques, and deliberate lifestyle adjustments are all necessary for navigating perimenopause and menopause. By promoting bone, heart, and mental health, these techniques not only assist reduce symptoms but also contribute to long-term wellness. Because every woman's experience is different, tailoring these strategies with the assistance of medical professionals can optimize the advantages.

PART TWO

3: Menopause

What Happens When Menstruation Ends

The end of a woman's reproductive years is signaled by menopause, a normal biological process that happens when the ovaries stop releasing eggs and menstruation permanently stops. Although the exact date might vary greatly, menopause is formally recognized when a woman has not had a monthly period for 12 consecutive months. This often happens between the ages of 44(early menopause) to 51 (normal menopause) to 55(late menopause).

The Menopausal Stages

Typically, menopause is broken down into three phases:

The period of transition before menopause, known as **perimenopause,** usually starts in a woman's late 30s or early 40s.

Menopause: The cessation of ovarian hormone production and fertility, indicated by the lack of menstruation for 12 months.

The phase following menopause is known as **post-menopause.**

Significance of Menopause as a Life Transition

Menopause marks a significant life shift; it shouldn't be seen as a sign of deterioration. Rather, it is a normal time when women may concentrate on taking care of themselves, changing their objectives, and accepting a new phase of their physical and mental health. After menopause, women can continue to have busy and satisfying lives by comprehending and controlling their symptoms.

Managing Menopause

A balanced diet, regular exercise, stress-reduction methods, and, in some situations, hormone treatment (MHT/HRT) are all part of a comprehensive approach to menopausal management. Women can be empowered to move through this time of life with support and resilience by being aware of the changes and having candid discussions with healthcare professionals.

Menopausal Symptoms No One Talks About

Menopause brings a range of symptoms that are often surprising and less frequently discussed, ranging from hair loss to strange skin sensations. Here are some of these symptoms, their possible hormonal origins, and how to manage them:

1. Menopausal Hair Loss

Symptoms include thinning hair, increased shedding, and even patchy hair loss.

Hormonal Causes: Low levels of progesterone and estrogen. Male-pattern baldness-like hair thinning patterns may increase if testosterone levels become more prevalent than estrogen.

Management:

Eat diets high in nutrients, especially zinc, biotin, and vitamins A, C, and E, will help maintain healthy hair.

Reducing stress and massaging the scalp to increase blood flow could also be beneficial.

Talk to your doctors about hormone replacement therapy (HRT) or think about topical therapies like minoxidil. For some, therapeutic massages or acupuncture provide comfort.

2. Frozen Shoulder

Characterized by pain, stiffness, and restricted shoulder range of motion.

Hormonal Causes: Since estrogen keeps joints flexible, low levels may trigger pain and inflammation, and reduced estrogen levels can cause stiffness in the joints and connective tissue, raising the risk of musculoskeletal problems like a frozen shoulder.

Management:

Anti-inflammatory diets, omega-3 supplements, and physical therapy exercises that preserve shoulder mobility are beneficial.

Therapeutic massages or acupuncture provide relief.

3. Weird Smells

Symptoms include an odd body odor and an enhanced or changed sense of smell.

Hormonal Factors: Sweat composition and production are affected by fluctuating estrogen levels, smell sensitivity and changes in body odor that may result from this. Changes in hormones can also affect the sense of smell, which leads to scents appearing more potent or distinct.

Management:

Using natural deodorants, staying hydrated, and dressing in breathable clothing can all be beneficial.

Eating whole plant-based meals lowers the smells connected to perspiration.

4. Insulin Resistance

Symptoms include cravings, elevated abdominal fat, blood sugar swings, and occasionally pre-diabetes.

Hormonal Causes: The body finds it more difficult to properly control blood sugar when estrogen levels are low because they decrease insulin sensitivity. This raises the risk of type 2 diabetes and causes weight gain, particularly in the abdominal region.

Management: Insulin sensitivity can be increased by eating a diet high in fiber and low in refined sugars, exercising often, and getting enough sleep.

Eat smaller, more frequent meals or intermittent fasting assists in normalizing blood sugar.

5. 3 A.M. Wake- Ups.

Hormonal Factors: Serotonin and melatonin (the hormones that control sleep) are released in response to fluctuations in estrogen and progesterone levels. These fluctuations make it difficult to get undisturbed, deep sleep.

Management:

Consider taking melatonin supplements and practicing excellent sleep hygiene, such as reducing screen time before bed.

Relaxing methods like progressive muscle relaxation or deep breathing can also be beneficial when attempting to get back to sleep,

6. Loss of Muscle

Symptoms include a loss of strength and muscular mass, frequently coupled with exhaustion.

Hormonal Factors: A decrease in testosterone and estrogen impacts muscle development and repair. Since estrogen indirectly promotes muscle building, its decrease can make maintaining muscle difficult, especially without consistent resistance training.

Management:

Eating enough protein and doing weight exercise regularly, is essential.

Maintaining muscular mass is aided by resistance training, such as body-weight exercises or weightlifting.

Omega-3 fatty acids and vitamin D also promote muscular health.

7. Body Fat/Visceral Fat

Symptoms include an increase in belly fat, especially around the waist.

Hormonal Causes: Increased visceral fat around the belly is frequently the result of altered fat distribution caused by lower estrogen levels. This fat has been linked to an increased risk of metabolic disorders and cardiovascular disease.

Management:

A diet low in processed foods and high in fibre and lean protein can aid in fat management.

Strength exercise and high-intensity interval training (HIIT) are particularly good in lowering visceral fat.

8. High Triglycerides and Cholesterol

Hormonal Causes: Estrogen controls the metabolism of fats consequently, a decrease in estrogen may raise triglyceride and cholesterol levels, raising the risk of heart disease.

Management:

Lowering saturated fats, eating heart-healthy fats (such as avocados and olive oil), and regular exercises can help lower cholesterol.

Red yeast rice and omega-3 supplements are beneficial for certain people.

9. Itchy Ears:

Symptoms: Sensitivity, dryness, and itching in the ear canal.

Hormonal Factors: Estrogen helps to keep skin supple and hydrated, so low estrogen levels can make the ear canal dry, which in turn makes it itchy and uncomfortable.

Management:

Avoid overcleaning, which can exacerbate dryness, and apply a mild moisturizer to the outer ear.

Adding moisture to the air using a humidifier might be beneficial.

10. Fatigue:

Symptom: Constant fatigue, even after getting enough sleep.

Hormonal Factors: Decreased levels of progesterone and estrogen impact energy production and sleep quality, resulting in fatigue. Disrupted sleep patterns and stress from menopausal symptoms also contribute to fatigue

Management:

Hydration, a healthy diet, and regular exercise are essential.

In addition to adaptogenic herbs like ashwagandha for stress resilience, B vitamins and magnesium can also help boost energy levels.

11. Anxiety

Symptoms include heightened stress, worry, and panic.

Hormonal Factors: Estrogen regulates dopamine and serotonin, which affect mood so increased anxiety, irritability, and stress sensitivity results from low estrogen levels.

Management:

Anxiety can be reduced by deep breathing, mindfulness, and meditation.

Natural supplements like magnesium or herbal medicines like St. John's Wort or valerian root (under a doctor's supervision).

12. Tinnitus (ear ringing)

Symptoms: A continuous buzzing or ringing sensation in the ears.

Hormonal Causes: Reduced estrogen affects blood flow and nervous system function, which can influence the inner ear and cause tinnitus. Additionally, stress and lack of sleep can make tinnitus symptoms worse.

Management:

Reducing caffeine intake and stress management

White noise machines or sound therapy

13. Dizziness

Symptoms include spinning sensations.

Hormonal Causes: Imbalances in the inner ear caused by changes in estrogen levels. Blood pressure changes during menopause also contribute to it.

Management

Blood pressure control, salt reduction, and vestibular exercises.

Staying hydrated.

14. Burning Tongue

Symptoms: A burning or tingling feeling in the mouth or tongue.

Hormonal Causes: Burning mouth syndrome, a frequent menopausal symptom, might result from lower estrogen levels that alter saliva production and nerve sensations in the mouth.

Management: Using mouthwash made for sensitive tongues

Avoiding hot or acidic meals, and drinking lots of water.

15. Crawling Sensations on the Skin

Symptoms include a crawling or itchy sensation beneath the skin.

Hormonal Causes: Low estrogen levels can cause formication, a painful "prickling" or "crawling" feeling that affects skin moisture and nerve endings.

Management: Applying cold lotions or creams and moisturizing often may help lessen the feeling.

Symptoms might also be lessened by cutting out on coffee and controlling stress.

16. Alcohol Intolerance

Symptoms include increased alcohol sensitivity, which can lead to unpleasant responses or faster intoxication.

Hormonal Causes:

Altered alcohol metabolism brought on by low estrogen and liver abnormalities. Additionally, alcohol exacerbates symptoms including sleep problems and heat flashes.

Management:

Maintaining a regular sleep pattern, engaging in cognitive activities, and remaining physically active.

For mental clarity, take diets high in omega-3 fatty acids, green tea, and blueberries.

17. Cognitive Fog (menopausal brain)

Symptoms include "fogginess," memory loss, and trouble focusing.

Hormonal Causes: estrogen promotes cognitive performance by influencing neurotransmitters like acetylcholine, which is involved in memory and learning.

Reduced amounts of estrogen can cause "brain fog," which impairs focus.

Management:

Maintaining a regular sleep pattern, engaging in cognitive activities, and remaining physically active.

For mental clarity, diets high in omega-3 fatty acids, green tea, and blueberries.

These symptoms demonstrate the wide range of effects that menopausal hormone changes may have on one's physical and emotional well-being. Knowing these might enable women to look for management techniques that work for them and are specific to their circumstances.

The impact of menopause on mental health.

Menopause frequently causes changes in mood, cognitive function, and emotional resilience, all of which can have a substantial impact on mental health. Hormonal changes, particularly the decrease in estrogen, which affects brain chemistry and neurotransmitter levels, are mostly to blame for these consequences.

1. Mood Swings and Emotional Health

Estrogen stabilizes mood by supporting neurotransmitters like serotonin and dopamine, which control emotional stability and well-being. When estrogen levels fall, these neurotransmitter levels may become unbalanced, increasing susceptibility to irritation, sadness, and anxiety.

Unpredictable Mood Swings and rapid emotional changes are common in some women in addition to sleep difficulties and physical discomforts like hot flashes and night sweats.

Sleep disturbances may particularly lead to a decreased emotional threshold, which makes it more challenging to control stress and preserve emotional equilibrium.

Stress and Life Transitions: Menopause frequently coincides with other major life transitions, such as children moving out or taking care of elderly parents, which can lead to more emotional stress when coupled with menopausal hormone changes, these stressors might heighten feelings of sadness, and frustration, or even loss of purpose.

2. Effects on the Brain

Menopause Brain or Cognitive Fog: Memory and concentration problems, sometimes known as "brain fog," are common among women. Estrogen is essential for maintaining cognitive function, particularly learning and memory formation. Reduced estrogen levels can cause these processes to malfunction, resulting in forgetfulness, trouble focusing, and a generalized sense of "fogginess."

Effect on Verbal Memory: Estrogen helps with verbal memory, which means that throughout menopause, it might become more difficult to remember names or words. In social or professional settings where verbal memory is crucial, this may be very annoying.

Menopausal cognitive fog is frequently temporary, but evidence suggests that women may be at slightly increased risk of cognitive deterioration in later life. Reading, social interaction, and cognitive exercises are common ways to keep the mind fresh before and after menopause.

In general, menopause can be difficult for mental health, but managing symptoms can be made simpler by knowing the underlying causes of these changes. For many women, maintaining a happy attitude and mental acuity during this transition can be facilitated by holistic techniques and expert support.

Tools for Coping

Menopausal symptoms can be managed by using hormone therapy, alternative therapies, and mindfulness exercises amongst others. Here is a summary of a few resources and tactics:

1. HRT, or Hormone Replacement Therapy

What It Is: Hormone replacement therapy (HRT) uses estrogen and progesterone supplements to compensate for the decline in hormones that occurs after menopause.

Benefits: Hot flashes, nocturnal sweats, vaginal dryness, and mood swings are just a few of the menopausal symptoms that hormone replacement therapy can help with. Additionally, it improves bone health by lowering the risk of osteoporosis.

Warning: Although HRT works for many people, it might not be appropriate for everyone. Talking with a healthcare professional is crucial to balancing the advantages and possible concerns because risks differ depending on a person's medical history.

2. Non-Hormonal Medications

Antidepressants: For those who are unable to utilize hormone replacement therapy, several antidepressants, especially SSRIs and SNRIs, can assist with mood swings and hot flashes.

Gabapentin: Often recommended to treat nerve pain, gabapentin has been shown to lessen night sweats and hot flashes, making it a non-hormonal therapy alternative.

Clonidine: Initially prescribed to regulate blood pressure, clonidine might also lessen hot flashes and enhance sleep quality.

3. Nutritional and Dietary Assistance

Phytoestrogens: Plant-based estrogens found in foods like soy, flaxseed, and legumes may alleviate some symptoms by slightly mimicking the effects of estrogen in the body.

Supplements: Supporting bone and muscle health with calcium, vitamin D, and magnesium is crucial for preventing the loss of bone density that comes with menopause. Additionally, fish oil's omega-3 fatty acids help promote brain function and potentially reduce mood swings.

Adaptogens: Herbal medicines such as Maca root, Rhodiola, and ashwagandha may help the body adjust to stress, which helps to enhance energy and sleep quality.

4. Stress-Reduction Techniques and Mindfulness Practices

Mindfulness Meditation: Being conscious as you meditate can help you manage stress, feel happier, and be more emotionally resilient. The awareness of bodily sensations and emotional reactions taught by meditation and mindfulness practices can be particularly helpful in managing hot flashes, anxiety, and irritation.

Yoga and Tai Chi: Research has demonstrated that gentle physical practices like yoga and tai chi can lessen menopausal symptoms including stress, anxiety, and even hot flashes. These exercises include breathing techniques, relaxation, and movement to support mental and physical health.

Breathwork: Deep breathing methods that soothe the nervous system, such as diaphragmatic or "box" breathing, might be helpful during hot flashes or increased stress.

5. Complementary and Alternative Medicines

Acupuncture: This age-old Chinese medicinal method has demonstrated potential in lowering mood swings, nocturnal sweats, and hot flashes. In addition to stimulating the body's natural painkillers and regulating energy flow, acupuncture may also balance hormonal reactions.

Hypnotherapy: Hypnosis can be useful in controlling symptoms, particularly those related to hot flashes. Hypnotherapy can help lessen the frequency and severity of hot flashes, by encouraging relaxation and assisting women in managing their reactions to stress.

6. Exercise

Aerobic Exercise: Walking, cycling, and swimming are examples of aerobic exercises that promote cardiovascular health and may alleviate some menopause symptoms like mood swings and anxiety.

Strength Training: Declining estrogen can influence bone density and muscle atrophy, which are counteracted by strength training. Additionally, resistance training increases metabolism and helps with weight control, which can be more difficult during menopause.

7. Keeping a Journal and Monitoring Symptoms

Symptom Diary: Women can monitor trends, pinpoint triggers (such as alcohol or caffeine), and assess the effectiveness of new therapies by keeping a record of their symptoms.

Emotional Processing: Journaling is a useful tool for managing the psychological changes that might come with menopause and for processing emotions.

Menopause management frequently calls for a mix of strategies. While some people find success with natural cures, lifestyle modifications, or mindfulness practices, others may benefit from hormone replacement therapy. Speaking with a healthcare provider can help tailor a plan that aligns with individual needs, promoting physical and mental well-being through this life phase.

Exercise for Muscle Maintenance

During menopause, some exercise techniques help maintain joint health, muscular development, and strength without overstimulating cortisol, the body's stress hormone. Excessive production of cortisol can cause tiredness, weight gain, and harm to muscles, so it's critical to approach exercise with recovery and balance in mind. Here are some specific workout suggestions:

1. Strength Training for Healthy Bones and Muscle Mass

Frequency and Intensity: Try to do two or three days of moderate-intensity strength exercise each week. Concentrate on compound exercises that target many muscular groups to support general strength without needing prolonged high-intensity sessions, such as squats, deadlifts, lunges, and rows.

Weight and repetitions: Use 8–12 repetitions for each set with modest weights, modifying according to comfort. This range increases stamina and strength without pushing the body to extremes, which can trigger cortisol release.

Exercise Types: Bodyweight, resistance band, and free weight exercises are great for joint health, especially for the knees and hips, because they don't put too much strain on the joints and provide a range of motion.

2. Low-Impact Cardiovascular Exercise

Walking and Cycling: Spend 20 to 30 minutes, three to five times a week, walking, riding, or swimming vigorously. Low-impact cardio increases metabolism, enhances circulation to joints, and promotes cardiovascular health without putting undue strain on the adrenal glands,

Interval Training: Without raising cortisol levels, low-intensity interval training, or LIIT, may be a useful strategy for preserving cardiovascular health. Switch between brief bursts of somewhat high-intensity activity (like rapid walking) and easy-to-moderate intensity (like walking).

3. Stretching and Mindful Exercise to Increase Joint Flexibility

Yoga: Yoga's slower, deliberate tempo helps regulate cortisol levels while combining strength and flexibility. Because they include strengthening and stretching poses that improve mobility, styles like Hatha and Yin yoga are especially good for joint health.

Pilates: Pilates helps stabilize the joints and promote muscular tone by emphasizing core strength, flexibility, and controlled motions. Its focus on deliberate, slow motions also reduces cortisol production.

Static Stretching: Adding static stretching at the end of exercises or as a stand-alone session improves muscular flexibility and relieves stress, which helps lessen tight joints.

4. Exercise with a Recovery Focus

Active Recovery Days: To aid muscle recovery and avoid cortisol accumulation from overtraining, schedule one or two days each week for low-intensity activities such as stretching, mild yoga, or a stroll.

Breathing Techniques: Deep breathing techniques, such as diaphragmatic breathing, can trigger the parasympathetic nerve system, which lowers cortisol and speeds up the healing process. Breathing can be performed at the end of a workout in addition to stretching or meditation.

5. Additional Tips for Minimizing Cortisol Production During Exercise

Avoid Overtraining: Prolonged, intense exercise can raise cortisol levels. Rather, concentrate on moderately intense, long-duration workouts, ideally lasting 30 to 45 minutes.

Ensure Adequate Recuperation: Give yourself at least 48 hours between strength-training sessions for the same muscle area, this will support muscle repair and help avoid excess cortisol release.

Post-Workout Nutrition: A modest intake of carbs and protein after exercise can promote muscle regeneration and lower cortisol.

These workouts promote muscle and joint health while maintaining appropriate cortisol production by balancing intensity and recuperation and combining several activities. Always listen to your body and modify your training regimen according to your feelings to create a fun and long-lasting habit.

Recommended Supplements

To promote bone health, hormonal balance, and general well-being, menopausal women are frequently advised to take supplements such as calcium, magnesium, vitamin D, and omega-3 fatty acids. The advantages of each are examined in further detail below:

1. Magnesium

Menopausal Benefits: Magnesium is necessary for energy generation, stress reduction, and muscle relaxation. Additionally, it can enhance the quality of sleep, which frequently deteriorates after menopause because of hormonal changes. Magnesium assists with symptoms like anxiety, mood swings, and even hot flashes because it supports the right balance of neurotransmitters.

Forms and Dosage: For people sensitive to other forms, Magnesium glycinate is a frequent form since it is generally well-tolerated and does not upset the stomach. Although 200–400 mg daily is advised, check with a healthcare provider for personalized advice.

2. Calcium

Benefits for Bone Health: Because low estrogen levels during menopause can cause bone density loss and raise the risk of osteoporosis, calcium is an essential element for strong bones. Vitamin D and calcium work well together to maintain bone mineral density.

Forms and Dosage: Consume 1,200 mg of calcium daily from diet and supplements. In contrast to calcium carbonate, calcium citrate is more easily absorbed and less harsh on the digestive tract.

3. Vitamin D

Beneficial Effects on Hormones and Bone Health: Vitamin D is essential for calcium absorption and bone health. Additionally, it boosts mood, physical strength, and immune function. Low vitamin D levels are associated with increased risks of heart disease, mental problems, and osteoporosis, so they are especially crucial during and after menopause.

Dosage and Sun Exposure: Take 600–800 IU daily (after consulting with your doctor), however, some people may require greater dosages, particularly if they don't get much sun exposure. The requirements for supplements can be evaluated by blood testing.

4. Omega-3 Fatty Acids

Benefits for Brain and Heart Health: Omega-3s, especially the anti-inflammatory EPA and DHA in fish oil, promote heart health, which is crucial because cardiovascular risk might rise after menopause. In addition to supporting cognitive function, which is frequently impaired by menopausal hormone changes, omega-3 fatty acids may also help reduce hot flashes and mood swings.

Dosage and Sources: A daily intake of 1,000 mg of mixed EPA and DHA is typical for overall health. Flaxseeds, fatty fish (such as salmon), and supplements containing fish or algal oil are good sources of omega-3 fatty acids.

Additional Considerations

A well-balanced diet full of vitamins, minerals, and antioxidants is the ideal combination for these supplements. Speaking with a healthcare professional is advised, to customize dosages and make sure there are no risky drug interactions,

When combined, magnesium, calcium, vitamin D, and omega-3 fatty acids provide a basis for hormonal balance, bone health, and general well-being during menopause.

Mental and Emotional Health

Using mental health resources, lifestyle changes, and social support can help manage mood swings, anxiety, and transitional experiences throughout menopause. Here's how each strategy might be beneficial:

1. Tools for Mental Health

Cognitive Behavioral Therapy (CBT): CBT helps people reframe negative beliefs and create healthy emotional reactions, which makes it a very useful tool for treating anxiety and mood swings. According to studies, cognitive behavioral therapy (CBT) helps menopausal symptoms by teaching coping mechanisms that might lessen emotional reactivity and boost resilience.

Meditation & Mindfulness: By focusing the mind on the here and now, mindfulness techniques like breathing and meditation can help lower stress and anxiety. Women who practice mindfulness are also better able to notice and accept their experiences without passing judgment, which might lessen the feelings of loss and change associated with menopause.

Journaling and Self-Reflection: Journaling offers a secure environment for processing feelings, reflecting on one's journey, and developing emotional intelligence. In addition to providing clarity, putting ideas and feelings on paper may highlight trends that improve mood swing management. Try using daily reflection or a gratitude notebook to recognize the good things in life even when things are changing.

2. Modifications in Lifestyle

Exercise: Regular exercise, including swimming, yoga, weight training, or walking, releases endorphins, which are naturally occurring mood enhancers that promote mental wellness. Additionally, exercise facilitates better sleep and helps control physical symptoms like hot flashes, which improves mental health.

Dietary Changes: Eating a well-balanced diet full of fruits, vegetables, whole grains, lean meats, and omega-3 fatty acids will help stabilize blood sugar and mood.

Additionally, foods high in tryptophan (found in turkey and eggs) and magnesium (found in leafy greens, almonds, and seeds) may help control anxiety and mood.

Sufficient Sleep: Getting enough sleep is essential for maintaining emotional balance. Sleep is crucial because it reduces anxiety and mood swings. Establishing a relaxing evening ritual, reducing the intake of alcohol and caffeine, and maintaining a regular sleep schedule can also enhance sleep quality.

3. Assistance from the Community

Participating in in-person or online menopausal support groups might offer emotional solace by allowing members to discuss their experiences. These groups may provide helpful advice for handling symptoms and emotions during this transition, promote connection and lessen feelings of isolation.

Therapeutic Communities: Online or local therapy groups centered on midlife transitions might offer a safe space for talking about difficulties related to menopause.

In addition to providing expert advice on coping mechanisms, group therapy may assist in normalizing feelings of loss.

Educational Workshops and Seminars: Women may gain knowledge and take charge of their health by attending webinars or seminars centered around menopause. Knowing the biological causes of worry and mood swings may be reassuring since it lessens emotions of confusion and frustration.

Practical Tips for Each Strategy

Create a Routine: Creating a daily schedule that includes specific periods for social interaction, exercise, and self-care can assist to maintain structure and regulate mood.

Limit Stressors: Saying no to too demanding obligations and relaxing will help reduce stress, which can boost mood and lower cortisol levels.

Practice Self-Compassion: Being nice to oneself and having patience will assist reduce self-criticism and aid in emotional adjustment during this difficult time of transition.

Together, these resources offer a thorough method for coping with the emotional shifts throughout menopause, promoting empowerment and overall well-being at every turn.

4: Post Menopause

Wellness, Longevity, and Life After Menopause

Overview of the Post Menopause Stage: Around a year following a woman's last menstrual cycle, she enters the post menopause stage, which is characterized by hormone stability, but at permanently lower levels. Since the ovaries no longer release eggs or generate appreciable amounts of the key reproductive hormones, estrogen and progesterone, these levels stay low. Here is a summary of the physical and hormonal changes that occur at this stage:

Hormone Balance After Menopause

Estrogen: Estrogen levels fall sharply and then level off. The ovaries no longer generate significant levels of estrogen in the absence of monthly cycles, while adipose tissue still produces trace amounts of the hormone. Numerous bodily systems are impacted by this change, such as skin elasticity, cardiovascular health, and bone density, because estrogen has preventive effects in these domains.

Similar to estrogen, the synthesis of progesterone decreases and stays low. After menopause, this hormone is no longer required because its main purpose is to get the uterus ready for conception. Low progesterone may affect mood and lead to worse sleep quality.

Testosterone: Although it is usually linked to male reproductive health, women can also make testosterone. During menopause, its levels steadily decrease, but they could stabilize beyond menopause. Women with low testosterone may have less libido and muscular mass.

Postmenopausal Physical and Emotional Changes

Bone Density: Women who have gone through menopause are more susceptible to osteoporosis since their estrogen levels are decreased. Because bone loss can occur more quickly, calcium, vitamin D, and weight-bearing exercise are essential for maintaining healthy bones.

Heart Health: A reduction in estrogen can raise the risk of heart disease after menopause since it protects cardiovascular health. A heart-healthy lifestyle that includes exercise, a well-balanced diet, and perhaps omega-3 supplements might be helpful.

Weight and Metabolism: Many women acquire weight, especially around the midsection, and have metabolic slowdowns. This might be connected to slower metabolic rates, reduced muscle mass, and altered insulin sensitivity.

Cognitive and Emotional Health: Hormonal fluctuations can also affect mood and cognitive performance. Low estrogen levels are associated with memory and processing speed issues, which are sometimes referred to as "menopause brain," even though mood swings typically lessen as hormone levels normalize.

Tips for Managing Postmenopausal Health

Keeping an active lifestyle, eating a healthy diet full of nutrients that support the heart and bones, and seeking support through healthcare guidance or community resources can help manage the challenges and support wellness in post menopause.

Women are more equipped to adjust to these changes and put their long-term health and well-being first when they recognize post menopause as a stage of life with new physiological standards.

Health Considerations unique to this stage; including bone density, cardiovascular health, and metabolism. Maintaining bone density, heart health, cognitive wellness, and sexual health during post menopause.

Key Supplements for Post menopause: Specific recommendations for vitamins, minerals, and adaptogens that help balance mood, boost energy, and support long-term health.

Adapting Exercise for Post menopause: Emphasis on strength training, flexibility exercises, and low-impact cardio to support aging joints, maintain muscle mass, and improve mental clarity.

Tips for Maintaining Wellness and Vitality through Diet, Exercise, and Self-Care Routines.

With regular exercise, healthy food, and self-care routines, it is possible to maintain health and vigor throughout menopause and beyond. Here are some useful pointers:

1. Dietary Strategies for Vitality

Focus on Nutrient-Dense Foods: Select foods high in vital minerals and vitamins. While magnesium and vitamin B promote energy and mental balance, calcium and vitamin D are crucial for bone health. Nuts, beans, fatty salmon, and leafy greens are all healthy options too.

Balance Proteins, Carbohydrates and Fats: To sustain energy levels and stable blood sugar, which can aid in mood regulation, aim for a balanced diet of macro-nutrients. Healthy fats (like avocado, olive oil, and almonds), lean proteins (like chicken, fish, and tofu), and complex carbs (such as whole grains, sweet potatoes and quinoa) support muscle maintenance and provide lasting energy.

Add Phytoestrogens: Plant-based estrogens in foods like soy, flaxseeds, and legumes can help reduce symptoms by imitating the body's natural estrogen. They can provide women with little hormonal assistance, but they cannot replace hormone treatment.

Drink enough water to assist digestion, enhance skin suppleness, and help regulate body temperature. Maintaining adequate hydration is crucial since it can reduce menopausal symptoms like dryness and bloating.

2. Exercise to Maintain Mental and Physical Health

Strength Training: Performing strength training activities two to three times per week will help maintain metabolic health, muscular mass, and bone density. In addition to supporting bone health and lowering the risk of osteoporosis, strength training can help reverse the natural muscle loss that occurs with ageing.

Cardiovascular Exercise: Low-impact cardio exercises that help control mood, promote weight loss, and enhance cardiovascular health include brisk walking, swimming, and cycling. Every week, try to get in at least 150 minutes of moderate-intensity exercise.

Flexibility and Balance Exercises: Pilates, yoga, or easy stretching techniques can help you stay flexible, avoid stiffness, enhance your balance, and reduce your chances of falling. Because they encourage relaxation and stress reduction, these exercises are also good for mental health.

Consistency over Intensity: The key is consistency. Select enjoyable and consistent activities, even if they are not strenuous. Frequent activity is more beneficial than short, intensive sessions.

3. Wellness Self-Care Practices

Prioritize Restful Sleep: Maintaining proper sleep hygiene is essential since menopause can affect sleep quality. Limit screen time before bed, create a relaxing evening routine, and stick to a regular sleep schedule. Stretching gently before bed or engaging in mindfulness exercises can also aid in mental relaxation.

Manage Stress with Mindfulness: Techniques like yoga, deep breathing, and meditation can assist in reducing stress, which promotes hormonal equilibrium and mental health. Journaling, artistic pursuits, and outdoor time can all help lower stress and improve mental clarity.

Establish Boundaries and Practice Self-Compassion: Embracing self-compassion helps enhance your emotional well-being and general perspective throughout the transitional period that is menopause. Setting limits on social or job commitments frees more time for self-care and personal development.

4. Make Use of Support Systems

Create a Helpful Community: Participate in menopause-related organizations or online discussion boards for support. It might be inspiring to know that you're not going through this shift alone, and it can provide understanding and a feeling of community.

Seek Professional Assistance When Needed: Experts in physical and mental well-being can offer individualized advice based on your requirements. Therapists, personal trainers, and nutritionists can assist you in creating a long-term strategy that suits your needs.

You can promote health and vitality during every phase of menopause by incorporating these suggestions into your everyday routine, improving your mental and physical health.

How Hormonal Changes Impact Brain Function, Memory, and Mood

Hormonal changes during menopause, particularly those involving estrogen, progesterone, and testosterone, can have a big impact on mood, memory, and brain function. Let's examine these hormones' effects on mental and emotional well-being in more detail:

1. Brain Function and Estrogen

Neuroprotective Role: Estrogen contributes to brain health by preserving neuron function and promoting cell division and repair. Additionally, it affects neurotransmitter systems critical for mood, memory, **and**

learning, including the dopamine and serotonin pathways.

Menopause-related declines in estrogen levels have been linked to alterations in memory and cognitive function, which are sometimes referred to as the "menopause brain." During perimenopause and menopause, many women experience problems with short-term memory, concentration, and cognitive speed. Estrogen supports the brain's hippocampus.

Estrogen reduction can impact the retention and recall of new information because estrogen supports the hippocampus (a part of the brain essential to memory processing).

2. Mood Regulation and Progesterone

Calming Effects: Progesterone works with the inhibitory neurotransmitter GABA (gamma-aminobutyric acid) to trigger relaxation, which calms the brain. Some women experience mood swings, sleep disturbances, and increased anxiety when their progesterone levels drop during perimenopause. This decrease may partially explain why mood swings are common during the transition, as the calming influence of progesterone wanes.

Sleep and Stress Resilience: By affecting GABA and cortisol, progesterone also promotes sound sleep. Because insufficient sleep is strongly associated with emotional instability and stress, low progesterone can interfere with sleep, making symptoms of exhaustion and mood swings worse.

3. Motivation and Testosterone

Drive and Confidence: Although women's testosterone levels are significantly lower than men's, this hormone affects mood, drive, and vitality. Commonly occurring after menopause, low testosterone levels can cause decreased libido, drive, and cognitive vigor. Motivation, vigor, and attention may all be significantly impacted by maintaining even low testosterone levels.

4. "Menopause Brain" and Cognitive Symptoms.

Memory: Some women have "brain fog" during menopause, which may manifest as forgetfulness or trouble focusing. The effects of reduced estrogen on the hippocampus (essential for memory formation and recall) are assumed to be the cause, though this is not true for all women.

Estrogen also impacts the prefrontal cortex, which controls mental clarity, decision making and processing speed. Lower levels can result in slower mental processing, which is often temporary but can feel disorienting.

5. Mood Swings and Emotional Changes

Anxiety and Depression: Because estrogen plays a major role in controlling serotonin levels (a neurotransmitter essential for mood stability) menopause may raise the risk of anxiety and depression. Some women may become more irritable, depressed, or even melancholy as a result of decreased serotonin activity.

Emotional Sensitivity: Women who experience hormonal fluctuations may become more emotionally reactive and sensitive to pressures. This emotional instability can be difficult, particularly when combined with menopausal physical symptoms like exhaustion and hot flashes.

Techniques for Managing Emotional and Cognitive Symptoms

Hormone replacement therapy, or HRT, can help some women manage their hormone levels and reduce symptoms that impact their mood, memory, and cognitive abilities. Talking with a healthcare professional about the advantages and disadvantages is crucial, though.

Lifestyle Changes: Maintaining mental health and mood throughout menopause requires regular exercise, a healthy diet, stress reduction, and good sleep hygiene.

Mental Exercises and Mindfulness: Learning new skills, practicing mindfulness, or participating in cognitive exercises can all assist maintain brain activity and enhance memory retention.

By being aware of these changes, women may take a proactive approach to their mental and emotional well-being by identifying and addressing the impacts of menopause on their cognitive and emotional health.

Evidence-Based Strategies and Techniques to "Resetting" the Menopause Brain

It is possible to optimize cognitive performance and emotional resilience during this period of life by "resetting" the menopausal brain with evidence-based methods in lifestyle modifications, cognitive training, and sleep optimization. These strategies promote general cognitive health and lessen the symptoms of "menopause brain,"

1. Modifications to Lifestyle

Frequent Exercise: Studies indicate that exercising regularly, particularly aerobic and resistance training, can improve mood, cognition, and brain function in general. Exercise promotes the production of neurotrophic factors, that promote neuron health, boosts blood flow to the brain, and can enhance the quality of sleep, which is essential for cognitive performance.

Anti-Inflammatory Diet: A diet high in antioxidants (found in vibrant fruits and vegetables), omega-3 fatty acids (found in fish, like salmon), and healthy fats (like olive oil and nuts), has been shown to support cognitive health. Specifically, omega-3 fatty acids are linked to better brain function and may lessen mood swings and brain fog brought on by menopause.

Stress Reduction Strategies: Prolonged stress raises cortisol levels, which over time may impair memory and emotional control. It has been demonstrated that yoga, breathing techniques, and mindfulness-based stress reduction (MBSR) can help control cortisol levels and enhance cognitive resilience by encouraging attention and relaxation.

2. Training of the Mind

Memory and Cognitive Exercises: Activities that promote neuroplasticity—the brain's capacity to rearrange itself and create new connections—include puzzles, memory games, and problem-solving exercises. Exercise for brain training can improve the neural networks responsible for executive function, memory, and attention.

Acquiring New Skills: Novel educational endeavors, like picking up a language, instrument, or pastime, have shown significant cognitive benefits. Novel learning encourages neurogenesis, or the growth of new neurons, particularly in the hippocampus, a part of the brain essential for memory and learning impacted by menopause.

Practices of Mindfulness and Meditation: Mindfulness meditation can enhance emotional stability, memory recall, and focus. A few weeks of mindfulness practice may improve cognitive flexibility and lessen age-related cognitive decline.

3. Optimizing Sleep

Sustaining Regular Sleep Patterns: The circadian rhythms of the body, which control sleep-wake cycles and promote restorative sleep, are synchronized by a regular sleep schedule. Cognitive clarity, mood stability, and memory consolidation depend on this regularity.

Practices for Sleep Hygiene: Sleep Quality can be enhanced by creating a peaceful and sleep-friendly atmosphere, particularly if menopause s

To improve the quality of your sleep, avoid using electronics right before bed, keep your room cold and dark, and practice relaxing techniques.

Magnesium and Melatonin Supplements: Research suggests that magnesium may promote relaxation and ease muscle tension, which can enhance the quality of sleep, while melatonin may assist in regulating sleep cycles, particularly for those going through hormonal changes.

Integrating these Strategies

Combining these strategies provides a cumulative effect that aids in "resetting" the menopausal brain by improving emotional resilience, mood stability, and cognitive clarity. By customizing these techniques to meet your unique needs, you can enhance mental health and make the menopausal transition easier to handle.

PART THREE

5: Managing Symptoms Naturally and Holistically

Natural Remedies and Lifestyle Changes That Can Help Relieve Symptoms.

Menopausal symptoms like mood swings, sleep difficulties, hot flashes, and more can be considerably managed with natural therapies and lifestyle modifications. These methods promote hormonal equilibrium, lowering inflammation, and enhance general health. Here are some successful tactics:

1. Modifications to Diet

- Phytoestrogens (present in plants like soybeans, flaxseed and legumes) are plant-based substances that can mimic the actions of estrogen in the body and may help reduce symptoms like hot flashes and night sweats.
- An anti-inflammatory diet that includes whole grains, fruits, vegetables, and foods high in omega-3 fatty acids (such as walnuts and salmon) can help to promote general health and lessen inflammation. This diet may help reduce fatigue, joint discomfort, and cognitive problems.
- Since menopause increases the risk of osteoporosis, Vitamin D and calcium are vital for

healthy bones. Leafy greens, dairy, and fortified foods are excellent sources.

2. Herbal Remedies

- A common remedy for hot flashes and night sweats is black cohosh. According to research, it might function via interacting with serotonin receptors.
- Evening Primrose Oil: Gamma-linolenic acid (GLA), present in evening primrose oil, may help control mood swings and breast pain.
- Maca Root: This is an adaptogen that may enhance mood and vitality and assist in balancing hormones.

3. Reducing Stress and Being Mindful

- Yoga and Meditation: Reduces stress, which can worsen menopausal symptoms. Specifically, yoga is known to enhance sleep quality and lessen hot flashes.
- Progressive Muscle Relaxation and Deep Breathing are two methods that help lower cortisol levels, which will lessen anxiety and promote calmness.

4. Exercise

- Aerobic Exercise: Consistent exercise helps minimize weight gain, ease hot flashes, and enhance mood.
- Strength Training: This is crucial for preserving bone density and muscle mass. Additionally, it aids in weight management, which may diffuse the intensity of symptoms.
- Flexibility Exercises: Techniques like Pilates and Tai Chi improve balance, ease stiffness, and encourage calmness.

5. Optimizing Sleep

- Practicing sleep hygiene tips like avoiding caffeine and alcohol before bed, setting up a consistent nighttime routine, and creating a cool, dark environment help optimize sleep. These actions enhance the quality of sleep, lowering mood fluctuations and weariness.
- Herbal Teas: Chamomile or valerian root teas can aid in promoting relaxation and improved sleep.

6. Massage and Acupuncture

- Acupuncture: Research indicates that promoting the nervous system, may lessen hot flashes and enhance general wellbeing.

- Massage therapy can help people feel happier, less stressed, and less tense.

7. Lifestyle and Hydration Adjustments

- Keep Yourself Hydrated: Drinking enough water might help with temperature control, bloating, and dryness.
- Limit Triggers: The frequency of hot flashes can be reduced by cutting back on alcohol, caffeine, and spicy meals.

8. Supplements to Help Manage Symptoms

- Omega-3 Fatty Acids: Promote stable mood and brain function. Present in flaxseed or fish oil
- Magnesium: Promotes better sleep, reduces anxiety, and muscular relaxation

9. Social Support and Mental Well-Being

- Join in Support Groups: Speaking with other menopausal women about your experiences can offer practical guidance and emotional support.
- Therapy or Counselling: It has been demonstrated that cognitive-behavioral treatment (CBT) improves emotional health and mood swings.

These natural therapies and lifestyle modifications are most effective when combined and customized to meet the needs of each individual. Speaking with medical experts can help guarantee the strategies selected to complement one's current health conditions and general health objectives.

Importance of Balanced Nutrition, Hydration, and Vitamins, Specifically Vitamins B, Magnesium, and Calcium.

Essential vitamins and minerals, enough hydration, and a balanced diet are key components in promoting general health and treating menopausal symptoms. Let's examine the significance of each, paying special attention to calcium, magnesium, and Vitamin B:

1. Balanced Diet: The Foundation of Menopausal Health

A well-balanced diet guarantees the body the nutrients it needs to support organ function, regulate hormone fluctuations, and sustain energy levels.

Benefits

Hormonal Balance: A diet high in complex carbs, lean proteins, healthy fats, and whole foods helps control hormone and blood sugar levels.

Weight control: Keeping a healthy weight lowers the chance of acquiring disorders like insulin resistance and heart disease, which can get worse after menopause.

Decreased Inflammation: Antioxidant-rich, nutrient-dense meals fight oxidative stress, which lowers inflammation and causes joint pains, mood swings and fatigue.

Cognitive Function: Memory and cognitive clarity may be impacted by B12 and folate deficiencies. Supplements can prevent "brain fog" and preserve brain health.

Energy Levels: B6 and B12 help produce red blood cells, which boost vitality and fight weariness.

Magnesium: The Mineral That Calms

Magnesium is essential for more than 300 enzymatic bodily functions such as nerve/muscle health and mood regulation.

Benefits

Stress and Sleep: Magnesium helps people relax and reduces the symptoms of anxiety and sleeplessness that are typical throughout menopause.

Together with calcium, bone health helps preserve bone mass and fend off osteoporosis.

Relaxing your muscles can help you avoid headaches, cramps, and spasms.

Calcium: The Basis for Healthy Bones

With declining estrogen levels, women are more susceptible to osteoporosis and bone loss during menopause.

Benefits

Bone Density: Calcium keeps bones healthy and helps keep them from breaking.

Heart Health: Supports the health of blood vessels and muscles, which contributes to cardiovascular function.

Muscular and Nerve Function: Assists in nerve transmission and muscular contraction, lowering the chance of cramping and numbness.

Practical Tips for Incorporating These Nutrients

Balanced Meals: Every meal should contain a range of fruits, vegetables, whole grains, lean meats, and healthy fats.

Choose fatty fish (omega-3s), legumes (vitamins B), and leafy greens (calcium and magnesium).

Hydration Practices: Drink eight glasses of water or more each day. Adapt to the degree of activity and the intensity of the symptoms.

Use herbal teas like chamomile, to increase hydration and lower anxiety.

Supplements (if required): To know if you require calcium, magnesium citrate, or Vitamin B-complex, speak with your healthcare professional.

In conclusion,

Menopause symptoms can be effectively managed with a balanced diet, enough water, and vital vitamins including calcium, magnesium, and B vitamins. They enable women to get through this stage with resilience and vitality by supporting everything from energy levels and cognitive clarity to bone density and mood stabilization.

Exercise and Relaxation Methods for Menopausal Health and Well-being

There are significant advantages to combining relaxation methods with physical activity like yoga and walking while treating menopause. These techniques help with problems including mood swings, hot flashes, sleeplessness, and cognitive fog, and they promote both mental and physical wellness. Here is an in-depth review of their effects and useful strategies:

1. Physical Exercise: Advantages and Methods

Yoga

Yoga incorporates consciousness, breathing techniques, and postures. It lowers stress chemicals like cortisol and increases strength, flexibility, and relaxation. Research indicates that it reduces anxiety, sleeplessness, and hot flashes.

Key Menopausal Poses:

- *Balasana (Child's Pose) soothes the mind and eases back pain.*
- *Bridge Pose (Setu Bandhasana): Eases fatigue and strengthens the spine.*
- *Legs Up the Wall Legs Up the Wall (Viparita Karani): Promotes better circulation and aids with sleep problems.*

Breathing Methods:

- *Nadi Shodhana, or alternate nostril breathing, calms the nervous system and reduces anxiety.*
- *Sheetali Pranayama, or cooling breath, helps control hot flashes by lowering body temperature.*

Strolling

This low-impact workout raises endorphin levels, improves mood, helps manage weight, and strengthens the heart. Additionally, regular walking helps lessen joint stiffness and enhance sleep.

Tips for Effective Walking: Try to walk for at least half an hour most days of the week.

- *Walk briskly to increase your heart rate or take leisurely walks outdoors to lower your stress levels.*
- *To increase your stamina and burn more calories, try interval walking, which alternates between rapid and moderate walking.*

Strength Training

Keeps up muscular mass, which typically declines as women go through menopause. Strength training lowers the risk of osteoporosis by increasing bone density.

Easy Workouts:

Increase strength without equipment by performing body-weight squats, lunges, and push-ups.

2. Relaxation Methods:

Meditation

Meditation lowers cortisol levels, encourages emotional equilibrium, and enhances mental performance. It works very well for controlling mood swings, anxiety, and sleep issues.

Simple Practice:

- *Locate a peaceful area, settle in, and spend ten to fifteen minutes concentrating on breathing.*
- *Beginners can maintain concentration through guided meditations (through apps or internet resources).*

PMR, or progressive muscle relaxation

- *Encourages relaxation and eases bodily strain.*
- *Each muscle group is tensed and subsequently relaxed during PMR, which is done gradually throughout the body.*

Mindful Breathing

- *It calms the mind and lowers stress by activating the parasympathetic nervous system.*
- *Practice the following: 4-7-8 Breathing: Take a deep breath for 4 counts, hold for seven counts,*

then exhale for eight counts. Repeat these four to five times.

3. Integrating Exercises for Maximum Well-being

- **Build a Routine:** *Add ten minutes of yoga or meditation to twenty minutes of walking.*
- **Be Consistent:** *Daily workouts, even if brief (10–15 minutes), are more successful than lengthier, irregular ones.*
- **Listen to Your Body:** *Adapt the intensity to your energy level and the intensity of your symptoms. Mild exercises are just as good as vigorous ones.*

Combining relaxation methods like meditation and mindful breathing with physical exercises like yoga and walking provides a comprehensive approach to menopausal management. They help women move through this period of life with grace and resilience by boosting physical strength, promoting emotional equilibrium, and improving general well-being.

Supplements and Herbs for Every Stage of Menopause

Vitamins, minerals, and herbal supplements can help manage menopausal symptoms naturally. During perimenopause, menopause, and postmenopause, these treatments help maintain hormonal balance, reduce common symptoms, and enhance general well-being.

1. Essential Minerals and Vitamins

Vitamin D

Role: Promotes immunological response, bone health, and calcium absorption.

Benefits include lowering the incidence of osteoporosis and reducing mood fluctuations.

Sources include supplements, seafood (such as salmon), sunlight, and fortified meals.

Calcium

Function: Essential for preserving bone mass.

Benefits: Prevents osteoporosis and bone loss, which are more prevalent after menopause.

Almonds, leafy greens, dairy products, and supplements are some sources.

Magnesium

Function: Controls mood, sleep, and the activity of muscles and nerves.

Benefits: Reduces muscular cramps, anxiety, and sleeplessness.

Sources: Whole grains, nuts, leafy greens and supplements like magnesium citrate.

Vitamins B12, B6, and B9

Function: Assist in regulating mood, cognitive activity, and energy production.

Benefits: Assist with mood fluctuations, cognitive problems, and exhaustion.

Sources: Fortified cereals, beans, leafy greens, eggs, and whole grains.

Omega-3 Fatty Acids

Role: Promote brain health and reduce inflammation.

Benefits include promoting cardiovascular health, lowering hot flashes, and improving emotional stability.

Sources: Supplements (fish oil or flaxseed oil), flaxseed, chia seeds, and fatty fish (mackerel, salmon).

2. Herbal Supplements

Black Cohosh

Function: Simulates the body's estrogen-like actions.

Benefits: Reduces mood swings, nocturnal sweats, and hot flashes.

Recommended Dosage: Available in capsule, liquid extract or tea form. Used as a 20–40 mg daily standardized extract.

Side Effects: Digestive upset, skin rashes, infection, muscle pain, breast pain /enlargement.

Evening Primrose Oil

Function: Contains the omega-6 fatty acid gamma-linolenic acid (GLA).

Benefits: Reduces mood swings, hot flashes, and breast soreness.

Dosage: 500–1,000 mg daily; frequently taken with vitamin E.

Side effects: Some people might get an upset stomach, diarrhoea, nausea and headaches.

Flaxseed

Role: A source of lignans, which are phytoestrogens.

Benefits: It naturally regulates estrogen levels, reducing hot flashes and elevating mood.

The recommended daily dosage is 1-2 tablespoons of ground flaxseed, with salads, yoghurt, or smoothies.

Maca Root

Function: An adaptogen that aids in the body's natural hormone balance.

Benefits: Enhances mood, libido, and vitality. Some women find it lessens hot flashes.

Dosage: Start by taking 1,500–3,000 mg of powder or capsules daily for up to 4 months.

Ashwagandha

Function: An additional adaptogen that lowers cortisol and stress levels.

Benefits include increased energy, better sleep, and assistance in managing anxiety.

Daily dosage: 300–500 mg standardized to at least 5% with anolides.

Red Clover

Red clover's function is as a phytoestrogen due to its isoflavone content.

Advantages: Could lessen hot flashes and improve heart health

Dosage: 40–80 mg of standardized extract each day.

3. Supplement Combination for Best Results

Flaxseed, Vitamin E, and black cohosh can work to manage hot flashes.

B-complex vitamins, magnesium, omega-3 fatty acids, and ashwagandha help stabilize mood.

Calcium, magnesium and vitamin D, work to promote healthy bones.

Magnesium + evening primrose oil + valerian root (optional) to promote sleep.

Safety Considerations

Before beginning supplements, speak with your healthcare provider, particularly if you are on medication or have underlying medical issues.

Quality Is Important: Select trustworthy brands to guarantee efficacy and purity.

Black cohosh, flaxseed, magnesium, and evening primrose oil are a few examples of herbs and supplements that provide natural solutions for managing menopausal symptoms at any stage. When paired with a healthy diet and way of living, they offer all-encompassing assistance for enduring menopause with resilience and vigor.

Diet and Nutrition: How to Balance Blood Sugar, Manage Weight, and Boost Energy Through Diet.

An important factor in controlling menopausal symptoms is diet. Stabilizing blood sugar levels, promoting good weight management, and sustaining energy levels throughout the day are all possible with a well-rounded strategy. Here's how to properly organize your diet:

1. Maintaining Blood Sugar Balance

Menopausal hormonal changes might impact insulin sensitivity therefore blood glucose control is crucial to preventing mood swings, exhaustion, and cravings.

Key Strategies:

- Give Low-Glycemic Foods Priority: Select carbs such as whole grains (quinoa, oats), legumes, and non-starchy vegetables that release glucose gradually.
- Mix Fiber, Protein, and Good Fats: Adding proteins or fats to carbs delays glucose

absorption. For instance, serve whole-grain toast with avocado or an apple with almond butter.

- Avoid Processed Sugars: Limit the refined sugars you consume from pastries, drinks, and white bread. These cause rapid spikes followed by crashes.
- Eat Balanced, Regular Meals: Frequent, little meals help keep blood sugar levels from falling. Eat balanced meals rich in protein, good fats, and complex carbohydrates.

2. Weight Management

Menopause-related weight gain is prevalent because of hormonal and metabolic changes. Here's how to properly manage it:

Key Strategies:

- Highlight Nutrient-Dense Foods: Eat a lot of nutritious grains, lean meats, veggies, and healthy fats. These offer vital nutrients without excess calories.
- Limit Portion Sizes: Be mindful of portions, particularly when consuming meals high in calories. Use smaller dishes or plates to reduce consumption.
- Lean proteins, such as those found in fish, tofu, or beans, can help preserve muscle mass and boost metabolism.

- Cut Down Processed Meals: Limit meals heavy in harmful fats and processed sugars, as these can contribute to weight gain and increase cravings.

3. Increasing Vitality

Menopause-related fatigue is common, but eating wisely might help you stay energized:

Key Strategies:

- Consume complex carbohydrates because they deliver energy gradually, unlike processed carbohydrates that produce crashes. Whole grains, legumes, and veggies supply this.
- Incorporate Foods High in Iron:
- Anemia is a contributing factor to tiredness. Add items such as lean red meat, lentils, and spinach.
- Hydrate Regularly: Fatigue might be mistaken for dehydration. Consume 8–10 glasses of water each day.
- Limit alcohol and caffeine: these substances can aggravate exhaustion and interfere with sleep cycles, even if they may give you a short-term boost.

Sample Meal Plans for Menopause Support

Meal Plan 1:

Breakfast: Have oatmeal with fresh berries, walnuts, and chia seeds, for fiber and long-lasting energy.

For Lunch: Quinoa salad with mixed greens, avocado, grilled chicken, and a lemon-tahini dressing for healthy fats and a well-balanced protein intake.

Snack: Greek yogurt paired with a tiny handful of almonds for some healthy fats and protein.

For Dinner: Baked salmon with steamed broccoli and sweet potatoes on the side for complex carbohydrates and omega-3 fatty acids.

Meal Plan 2: Mediterranean-Style

Greek yogurt topped with walnuts, flaxseeds, and honey for breakfast.

Lunch consists of quinoa and chickpea salad topped with cucumber, feta, cherry tomatoes, and olive oil.

Dinner will be baked fish served with wild rice and steamed asparagus.

Meal Plan 3: Hormone Balancing

Breakfast consists of chia seed pudding with almond milk and fruit on top.

Lunch consists of grilled chicken, sweet potato mash, and greens.

Dinner will be brown rice, bell peppers, broccoli, and stir-fried tofu.

Meal Plan 4: High Protein Boost

Breakfast is whole-grain bread with scrambled eggs, avocado, and spinach.

Lunch is a whole wheat tortilla wrapped with turkey and avocado.

Dinner will be a lentil stew with kale, carrots, and onions.

Meal Plan 5: Anti-Inflammatory Diet

Smoothie with banana, spinach, almond butter, and unsweetened almond milk for breakfast.

Lunch: Mixed greens, salmon, avocado, and lemon dressing.

Dinner will include grilled chicken, quinoa seasoned with turmeric, and roasted cauliflower.

Meal Plan 6: Plant-Based Option

Breakfast consists of overnight oats, mango, chia seeds, and almond milk.

Lunch is a dish of black beans and quinoa accompanied with salsa and avocado.

Dinner will be tomato basil sauce over zucchini noodles with tofu.

Meal Plan 7: Foods That Give You More Energy

Breakfast: Blueberries, pumpkin seeds, and oatmeal with walnuts toppings.

Lunch is a bed of spinach with tuna salad dressed with olive oil.

Dinner: Baked fish served with sweet potato wedges and roasted Brussels sprouts.

Meal Plan 8: Focus on Bone Health

Breakfast consists of almonds, pineapple, and cottage cheese.

Lunch consists of arugula salad and sardines served on whole-grain crackers.

Dinner will be a stir-fried chicken and broccoli with sesame seeds and brown rice.

Meal Plan 9: Blood Sugar Balance

Avocado, veggies, and scrambled tofu for breakfast.

Lunch will be a dish of black beans and brown rice with guacamole.

Dinner is quinoa, steaming green beans, and grilled shrimp.

Meal Plan 10: Weight Management Focus

Breakfast consists of cherry tomatoes, whole-grain bread, and hard-boiled eggs.

Lunch is a salad of spinach and lentils dressed with lemon tahini.

Dinner will include roasted sweet potatoes, greens, and baked turkey breast.

Rich in whole foods, lean proteins, healthy fats, and complex carbohydrates, these meal plans are perfect for promoting hormonal balance, lowering inflammation, and increasing energy levels throughout menopause.

It is possible to efficiently stabilize blood sugar, manage weight, and increase energy throughout menopause by eating a balanced diet full of whole foods, lean proteins, healthy fats, and low-glycemic carbohydrates. Healthy eating practices, water, and nutrient-dense foods lay the groundwork for flourishing during this change.

Stress Management

Managing Stress During Menopause: Preventing Increases in Cortisol

The "stress hormone," cortisol, can increase during menopause as a result of hormonal changes, which can lead to mood swings, exhaustion, and weight gain. Effective stress management is essential to preventing these increases and advancing general well-being. Here are some helpful strategies:

1. Mindfulness Practices

Because mindfulness focuses on the here and now, it decreases cortisol levels, reducing stress.

Frequent meditation, even for just five to ten minutes each day, can dramatically lower anxiety and cortisol levels.

Body Scan Meditation: Release stress by focusing on several body parts one after the other.

Walking mindfully: Walking deliberately and slowly while taking in your environment helps you de-stress and ground yourself.

2. Breathing Exercises

Breathing control triggers the parasympathetic nervous system, reducing stress:

Diaphragmatic (Belly) Breathing: Find a comfortable position to sit or sleep in. Put a hand on your tummy and another on your chest.

Breathe deeply through your nose, letting your diaphragm expand so that your belly, not your chest, rises.

Breathe out slowly through your lips. For five to ten minutes, repeat.

The 4-7-8 Breathing Technique involves four seconds of inhalation, seven seconds of holding, and eight seconds of exhalation.

Tip: Practice these techniques during stressful moments or before bed to enhance relaxation.

3. Mild Exercise

While high-intensity exercises might momentarily raise cortisol, exercise gradually lowers it. Activities that are steady and gentle are best:

Yoga: Enhances strength and flexibility while lowering stress by combining movement and awareness.

Particularly soothing poses are savasana, cat-cow, and child's pose.

Low-impact activities like swimming or walking might help you decompress and reduce stress without overtaxing your adrenal glands.

Tai Chi and Qigong are age-old techniques that focus on deep breathing and slow, deliberate motions that are proven to relax the nervous system.

4. Modifications to Lifestyle

Habits can help control cortisol levels:

Maintain a Regular Sleep Schedule: Sleep deprivation raises cortisol levels. .

Balanced Diet: Avoid excess sweets and coffee since these might raise cortisol levels.

Reduce screen time: Limit screen time, particularly just before bed. Stress is exacerbated by blue light and constant alerts.

5. Creative and Calm Activities

Taking part in your favorite pastimes or activities can lower cortisol levels. Reading, listening to music, or gardening are all hobbies that increase dopamine and serotonin, which balance cortisol.

6. Muscle Relaxation Progressively (PMR)

By tensing and releasing various muscle groups, this approach helps relieve physical stress associated with cortisol increases.

Methods for Practice:

Tense your muscles for 5–10 seconds, then relax them, starting with your feet.

Proceed through your body, starting with your arms, face, chest, belly, thighs, and calves.

7. Restrict Your Use of Stimulants

Reduce consumption of alcohol and caffeine as these raise cortisol levels. Instead of coffee, use herbal teas with relaxing properties, like peppermint or chamomile.

8. Support and Social Connection

Getting involved with friends or support groups might help you feel less stressed and alone. Cortisol levels are normally lowered by laughter and deep relationships.

By implementing these methods into your daily routine, you may greatly lower stress levels, support hormonal balance, and enhance your general well-being throughout menopause.

6: Hormone Replacement Therapy (HRT) and Other Medical Options

Overview:

First, what is HRT or hormone replacement therapy?

Hormone supplements, usually estrogen and occasionally progesterone, are used in hormone replacement therapy (HRT) to treat menopausal symptoms such as vaginal dryness, mood swings, hot flashes, and night sweats. It eases the body's transition by bringing hormone levels back to levels seen before menopause.

Advantages of HRT

Symptoms Relief: It lessens vaginal dryness, hot flashes, and nocturnal sweats.

Bone Health: By preserving bone density, it reduces the chance of osteoporosis.

Mood and Cognitive Support: According to ongoing studies, this may help lessen mood swings and lower the risk of dementia.

Considerations and Risks

HRT isn't suitable for everyone long-term usage may raise several hazards, especially:

Long-term usage of EPT may marginally increase the risk of breast cancer.

Blood clots and strokes are more likely to occur with oral HRT, while they are less likely with transdermal patches.

Heart Disease: Women with pre-existing cardiovascular conditions should not use HRT.

Tip: The risks differ according to the kind of HRT, age, and medical history. Consult a healthcare professional about your alternatives in detail.

Other Options

There are several medical options available to women who cannot or do not want to use HRT:

A. SSRIs, or Selective Serotonin Reuptake Inhibitors

- *Use: Low dosages can aid in managing mood swings and hot flashes.*
- *Examples include Paroxetine (Brisdelle) and Venlafaxine (Effexor).*

b. Gabapentin

- *Good for night sweats and hot flashes.*
- *Off-label usage of this anti-seizure drug for menopausal symptoms has increased.*

c. Clonidine

- *Use: Reduces hot flashes and lowers blood pressure.*
- *Form: Available as a skin patch or tablet.*

d. Vaginal Estrogen

- Addresses localized symptoms such as atrophy and *dryness of the vagina.*
- *Forms: Rings, pills, or creams.*

Complementary Healthcare Services

- *Acupuncture can lessen hot flashes and enhance sleep quality.*
- *Cognitive Behavioral Therapy (CBT): Assists in managing stress, anxiety, and mood fluctuations.*

The therapeutic selection is based on: Symptom severity, medical history (personal and familial) and personal preferences for medical versus natural remedies.

Important Tip: When using hormone replacement therapy or any other medical treatment for menopause, frequent checkups are essential.

Though not the sole choice, HRT can greatly enhance the quality of life throughout menopause. Understanding the spectrum of medical and complementary therapies enables you to make a well-informed choice that suits your requirements.

HRT Types and Their Effects

1. Estrogen Therapy (ET)

- The main goal is to treat symptoms brought on by an estrogen shortage.
- Night sweats and hot flashes: ET lessens the occurrence and intensity of vasomotor symptoms.
- Dry vagina: Local estrogen therapies (rings, lotions) bring back suppleness and moisture.
- Bone Health: It prevents osteoporosis by preserving bone density.
- Forms include vaginal treatments, topical gels, transdermal patches, and oral tablets.
- Ideal For: Women without a uterus who have had a hysterectomy.

2. Combined Estrogen- Progesterone Therapy (EPT)

- Its function is to shield the uterine lining against hyperplasia, or expansion, caused solely by estrogen.
- Mood and Emotional Well-Being: Progesterone can help control fluctuations in mood.

- Sleep Disruptions: Progesterone helps some women sleep better by calming them down.
- Forms: Combination creams, patches, or oral tablets.
- Ideal For: Women whose uteruses are still intact.

3. Testosterone Supplements

- Less frequently used, although it serves to address:
- Low Libido: May increase libido and vitality.
- Fatigue and Muscle Loss: Supports the preservation of physical strength and muscle mass.
- Form: Usually patch or cream formulations.
- Note: It requires close monitoring because of possible adverse effects,

How Certain Symptoms Are Addressed by HRT

Night sweats and hot flashes:

- *This is brought about by estrogen withdrawal, which impacts the hypothalamus, which controls body temperature.*
- *Treatment: The most successful method for lowering frequency and severity is systemic estrogen treatment.*

Dryness and atrophy of the vagina:

- *This happens as a result of the vaginal tissues being thinner and less elastic.*
- *Treatment: With little systemic absorption, localized estrogen (cream, ring) offers focused relief.*

Depression and Mood Swings:

- *This is associated with changes in progesterone and estrogen levels that impact neurotransmitters such as serotonin.*
- *Therapy: HRT in combination with low-dose antidepressants*

Bone Loss (Osteoporosis)

Bone density loss is accelerated by estrogen deprivation.

Alternatives for women who are unable to take HRT include:

- *SSRIs, gabapentin, and clonidine are among the medications used to treat symptoms.*
- *Supplements: Vitamin E, flaxseed, and black cohosh may provide some minor relief.*
- *Lifestyle Interventions: Stress reduction, exercise, and diet all have a big influence on symptom control.*
- *Knowing how hormone fluctuations affect symptoms gives women the ability to select the*

best course of action for their particular requirements.

- *Treatment: Bisphosphonates or selective estrogen receptor modulators (SERMs) are alternatives to estrogen treatment.*

Sleep Disruptions

- *Which might be frequently brought on by hormone abnormalities and nocturnal sweats.*
- *Treatment options include lifestyle modifications and sleep hygiene techniques, as well as progesterone's potential soothing effects.*

Cognitive Symptoms ("Menopause Brain")

- *Neurotransmitter activity and brain function are impacted by estrogen.*
- *Treatment: Although studies are still being conducted, several women claim that HRT improves their cognitive function.*

Selecting the Appropriate Care

- **Customized Approach:** HRT should be customized based on a woman's unique symptoms, medical background, and risk factors.
- **Duration and Dosage:** To reduce hazards, use the lowest effective dose for the shortest time.

- **Monitoring:** Routine follow-ups are crucial, to evaluate the advantages and drawbacks.

HRT Substitutes

- Alternatives for women who are unable to take HRT include:
- SSRIs, gabapentin, and clonidine are among the medications used to treat symptoms.
- Supplements: Vitamin E, flaxseed, and black cohosh may provide minor relief.
- Lifestyle Interventions: Stress reduction, exercise, and diet all have a big influence on symptom control.

Knowing how hormone fluctuations affect symptoms gives women the ability to select the best course of action for their particular requirements.

Tips for Having Knowledgeable Discussions with Medical Professionals During Menopause

Although navigating menopause can be challenging, having candid, educated discussions with medical professionals can help customize treatment regimens to meet your specific requirements. Here's how to maximize these conversations:

1. Get everything ready in advance

- *Track Your Symptoms: To spot trends, keep a symptom log that includes mood swings, heat flashes, and sleep disturbances.*
- *List your worries: Prioritize inquiries concerning alternate alternatives, side effects, and remedies.*
- *Know your history: List your current prescriptions, dietary supplements, and family medical history, particularly those relating to osteoporosis or breast cancer.*

2. Educate Yourself

- *Know the Fundamentals of Menopause: Learn about words such as post menopause, perimenopause, and hormone replacement therapy.*
- *Research Options: To be able to talk about them, educate yourself on both hormonal and non-hormonal therapy.*

3. Be Specific and Honest

- *Share All Symptoms: Even seemingly unrelated symptoms, such as mood swings or memory problems, may be significant.*
- *Talk about lifestyle factors: Decisions about therapy may be influenced by your stress levels, exercise regimen, and nutrition.*

4. Seek clarification and ask questions

Some examples of important questions are:
- *"What are the advantages and disadvantages of hormone replacement therapy for my particular situation?"*
- *Ask about Alternatives*
- *Ask about the long-term Impact*

5. Examine Tailored Treatment Programs

- *Personalized Approach: Ask for a strategy specific to your symptoms, way of life, and health risks.*
- *Frequent Check-Ins: Talk about the necessity of follow-up consultations to track development and modify treatments as needed.*

6. Openly Address Risks and Benefits

- *Recognize trade-offs: There are hazards associated with every therapy. Be sure you comprehend any possible adverse effects and how they stack up against untreated symptoms.*
- *Obtain a Second Opinion: Do not be afraid to seek clarification from another medical expert if you are unclear.*

7. Ask About Examinations and Evaluations

- *Hormone Levels: Find out if testing for hormones (such as FSH and estrogen) is required to direct treatment.*

- *If you are susceptible to osteoporosis, bone density tests are essential.*

8. Bring Support

- *Go with a Companion: Having a friend or family member with you might support you emotionally and aid with memory recall.*
- *Make Notes: Jot down important topics throughout the meeting so you may review them later.*

9. Make Use of Available Resources

- *Request Suggestions: Ask for information or reading materials to help you better comprehend your therapy.*
- *Explore Support Groups: Your provider may recommend local or online menopause support communities.*

10. Speak Up for Yourself

- *Trust Your Instincts: If you feel ignored, don't be afraid to look for another healthcare practitioner who will listen to your worries.*
- *Collaborative Approach: Keep in mind that you are more than simply a patient; you are a partner in your healthcare.*

Through careful preparation and active participation, you will enable yourself to make well-informed decisions on the optimal management of menopause.

7: Hormones, Sexual Health, and Intimacy After Menopause

Sexual Health and Menopause: The Impact of Hormonal Changes on Libido, Vaginal Health, and Arousal.

1. Changes in Hormones During Menopause

The levels of hormones, especially estrogen and testosterone, are drastically changed after menopause, impacting several facets of sexual health:

a. The decline in estrogen:

- *Health of the Vagina: Vaginal atrophy, or the weakening, dryness, and inflammation of vaginal tissues, is caused by low estrogen levels. This may result in:*
- *Dryness of the vagina*
- *Pain or discomfort during sexual activity (dyspareunia)*
- *Decreased suppleness of the vagina*
- *Arousal and Libido: Blood flow to the pelvic area is partly maintained by estrogen. Declining sensitivity might make arousal more challenging.*

b. Decline in Testosterone:

- *Despite being mainly linked to men, testosterone also affects women's energy, libido, and sexual arousal.*
- *Impacts: Lower levels may lead to:*
- *Reduced lust for sex*
- *Diminished intensity of orgasm*
- *Overall exhaustion and diminished drive*

2. The Effects of These Modifications on Sexual Health

a. Sexual Drive, or Libido:

- *Reduced interest in sex can result from lower levels of estrogen and testosterone.*
- *Psychological Factors: Menopause may be accompanied by mental disorders (depression, anxiety) or life changes (empty nest, relationship changes), all of which have an impact on libido.*

b. Health of the vagina:

- *Dryness and atrophy of the vagina: Less lubrication and suppleness might cause pain or discomfort during sexual activity.*
- *pH Shifts: Reduced estrogen levels can change the microbiome in the vagina, raising the risk of infections (such as vaginal infections and urinary tract infections).*

c. Orgasm and Arousal:

- *Reduced Blood Flow: Less estrogen affects the vaginal region's blood flow, which might lessen sensation.*
- *Clitoral Alterations: Arousal and orgasmic response may be impacted by a less sensitive clitoris.*

Treatment Options: Vaginal Dryness, Discomfort, and Reduced Libido

Hormonal changes, particularly the decrease in estrogen and testosterone, are mostly responsible for menopausal symptoms such vaginal dryness, pain, and decreased libido. A mix of medical interventions, home cures, and lifestyle changes are frequently used to address these issues.

1. Health Care Services

a. Vaginal Estrogen Therapy

- *Types: Comes as suppositories, pills, rings, and creams.*
- *How It Operates: improves lubrication and decreases atrophy by delivering low-dose estrogen directly to vaginal tissues without having a major effect on total hormone levels.*
- ***Examples***
- *Estrace (Cream)*
- *Vagifem (Tablet)*
- *Estring (Ring)*

b. Systemic Hormone Replacement Therapy (HRT)

- *Use: For more general menopausal symptoms, such as decreased libido and dry vagina.*
- *Forms: implants, gels, patches, or pills.*
- *Considerations: Talk to a medical professional about balancing the advantages and disadvantages (e.g., breast cancer, cardiovascular concerns).*

c. Testosterone Therapy

- *Function: Assists with low energy and libido.*
- *Application: Because too much testosterone might have negative consequences like acne or hair growth, it is frequently used in combination with HRT under medical supervision.*

d. Ospemifene (Osphena)

- *Use as an oral drug that relieves painful sex by acting in vaginal tissues similarly to estrogen.*
- *Who It's For: Women who have gone through menopause and are unable or unwilling to undergo estrogen treatment.*

2. Alternatives to Hormonal Medicine

a. Moisturizers and Lubricants

- *Lubricants: Offer momentary comfort during sexual activity.*
- *Types include oil-based (which could not work with condoms), silicone-based (which lasts longer), and water-based (like KY Jelly).*
- *Moisturizers: Continue to hydrate.*
- *Examples include natural alternatives like coconut oil or Replens.*

b. Prasterone or Dehydroepiandrosterone (DHEA)

- *Form: implant for the vagina.*
- *Benefit: Promotes the body's natural synthesis of estrogen, improving the health of vaginal tissue.*

3. Organic Remedies and Supplements

a. Black Cohosh

- *Use: Traditionally used to treat menopausal symptoms, this medication may mitigate vaginal dryness indirectly by regulating hormone levels in the body.*

Note: *Due to potential liver issues, consult a doctor.*

b. Flaxseed

- *Benefit: Contains phytoestrogens, which are estrogens derived from plants, which may help reduce dryness.*

c. Vitamin E

- *Application: Some women apply vitamin E oil straight to the tissues of their vaginas.*

d. Omega-3 Fatty Acids

- Source: Flaxseed oil and fish oil.
- Benefit: Aids in preserving the health of vaginal tissues and other mucous membranes.

4. Behavioral and Lifestyle Methods

a. Regular Intercourse or Intimation

- *Benefit: Maintains suppleness by improving blood flow to vaginal tissues.*
- *A vaginal dilator might be helpful if having sex is unpleasant.*

b. Kegel exercises for the pelvic floor

- *Use: To increase blood flow and improve sexual function, strengthen the muscles in the pelvis.*

c. Hydration and Nutrition

- *Focus: Whole grains, leafy greens, and meals high in omega-3 fatty acids (like salmon) promote tissue health and hormonal balance.*
- *Hydration: Drinking enough water keeps the body and vaginal tissues from being dehydrated.*

5. Handling Decreased Libido

a. Methods of Mindfulness and Relaxation

- *Practice: Yoga, meditation, and deep breathing techniques help people cope with stress, a cause of low libido.*

b. Counseling and Communication

- *Importance: Psychological problems impeding intimacy can be addressed by psychotherapy (such as sex therapy) and open communication with a partner.*

Menopausal vaginal dryness, pain, and decreased libido are frequently best relieved by a multifaceted strategy that includes medication therapies, natural remedies, and lifestyle modifications. Working with a healthcare professional guarantees a customized treatment plan that fits your preferences and health requirements.

The Importance of Open Communication, Self-Compassion, and Redefining Intimacy in Menopause

1. Communicating Openly with Partners

Why It Matters: Menopause may cause major changes in the body, mind, and emotions, which affects relationships and intimacy frequently. An open line of communication strengthens the bond between spouses by promoting understanding and support.

Key Benefits:

- *Improves Understanding: Talking about symptoms like mood swings, exhaustion, or decreased libido makes it easier for partners to understand the difficulties.*
- *Minimizes Misunderstandings: Sincere communication helps to avoid misunderstandings about behavioral changes and promotes empathy.*
- *Encourages Joint Solutions: By discussing their emotions and worries, couples may look for methods to be close and intimate, whether that means changing their way of life or finding new ways to be intimate.*

Practical Tips:

- *Plan Talks: Select peaceful times to have conversations, concentrating on feelings rather than assigning blame.*
- *Make use of "I" statements: Instead of projecting thoughts like "you don't understand me," express your feelings like "I feel tired."*

- *Encourage Involvement: Encourage partners to voice their thoughts and include them in learning about menopause.*

2. Compassion for Oneself

Why It Matters: Because of the physical changes and social constraints associated with aging, menopause frequently causes feelings of loss or dissatisfaction. Self-compassion exercises promote emotional health and resilience.

Key Aspects:

- *Accept Change: Acknowledge menopause as a normal stage rather than a deterioration. Move away from self-criticism and toward acceptance.*
- *Practice Self-Care: Putting one's physical, mental, and emotional well-being first strengthens one's sense of value.*
- *Challenge Negative Thoughts: Swap out harsh self-evaluations with affirmations on your resilience and strength.*

Practical Tips:

- *Daily Affirmations: Remind yourself of your worth and strengths, which go beyond appearances.*

- *Mindfulness Practices: Methods such as meditation foster self-awareness and self-compassion.*
- *Establish Boundaries: Give priority to enjoyable activities and limit stressful commitments.*

3. Redefining Intimacy

The significance of menopause lies in the chance it presents to delve into more profound and significant types of connection that go beyond conventional sexual engagement. This change may result in a stronger sense of fulfilment and emotional connection.

Expanding the Meaning of Intimacy

- *Emotional Closeness: Relationships are strengthened when worries, hopes, and experiences are shared.*
- *Physical Affection: Non-sexual contact, such as massage, hand holding, or snuggling, may keep people close.*
- *Shared Activities: Taking part in pastimes or novel experiences together strengthens bonds.*

Adjustments for Sexual Intimacy:

- *Exploration: Try out novel approaches to happiness and contentment.*
- *Put Connection First: Prioritize enjoyment for both parties above performance.*

- *Seek Support: Tools for managing changes together can be obtained via counselling or sex therapy.*

Couples may successfully endure menopause as a transforming, bonding experience by practicing open communication, self-compassion, and a broader definition of intimacy. Discovering a new depth and kinship beyond this period of change promotes comprehension and adjustments resulting in a flourishing partnership.

Menopause Symptom Scoring Sheet (The Greene Scale): Tracking Symptom Severity and Spotting Patterns

The Greene Climacteric Scale: What is it?

A validated instrument for gauging the intensity of menopausal symptoms is the Greene Climacteric Scale. Created by Dr. Jeremy Greene, this self-assessment tool assists women in monitoring their vasomotor, psychological, and physical symptoms during menopause, helping medical professionals understand how symptoms develop and how well therapies work.

The Greene Scale's components include:

There are three primary symptom categories on the scale:

Psychological Signs and Symptoms:

- *Anxiety: Nervousness, stress, and panic attacks*
- *Depression: Mood swings, sobbing fits, and a depressed state*

Somatic (physical) symptoms

- *Headaches, joint and muscle discomfort.*
- *Sleeping difficulties*
- *Exhaustion*

Vasomotor symptoms

- *Night sweats and hot flushes.*

Every symptom is graded according to its intensity:

- *0 = Not at all*
- *1 = A little amount;*
- *2 = A significant amount*
- *3 = Highly*

How the Greene Scale Is Used:

1. Self-Evaluation:

- *Fill out the survey on a weekly or monthly basis.*
- *Give each symptom an honest rating depending on how it affects day-to-day living.*

2. Track Patterns:

- *Identify patterns over time, such as heightened symptom severity.*
- *Identify factors that impact the intensity of symptoms, such as dietary changes, stress, or sleep patterns.*

3. Communicate with Medical Professionals:

- *The information offers a clear picture of how symptoms develop,*
- *supports the customization of treatment regimens, whether they involve medication, alternative cures, or lifestyle modifications.*

4. Assess the efficacy of treatment:

- *Scores before and after starting treatments (HRT, vitamins, etc.) should be compared.*
- *Interventions should be modified in response to shifts in symptom severity.*

Advantages of the Greene Scale:

- *Empowerment: Boosts self-awareness and health-related control.*
- *Objective Data: Offers quantifiable information for medical consultations.*
- *Personalized Care: Encourages treatment regimens specific to each patient's symptoms.*

Practical Tips:

- *The Key Is Consistency: To ensure reliable comparisons, complete the scale at the same time of day.*
- *Note your lifestyle factors: Note stress, nutrition, and exercise alongside scores for a comprehensive picture.*

Through consistent use of the Greene Climacteric Scale, women may actively track their menopausal journey and make sure they get the best care and support for their particular circumstances.

Hot Flash Diary and Symptom Journal:

A Hot Flash Diary and Symptom Journal: What Is It?

Women keep detailed records of their menopause-related symptoms, especially hot flashes, in a Hot Flash Diary or a Symptom Journal. It assists in determining trends, causes, and the efficacy of therapies or lifestyle modifications. Women who maintain a thorough diary can control their symptoms better and give medical professionals insightful information for individualized treatment.

Its contents include:

Symptom Record:

- *Date and Time: Note the occurrence of each symptom.*
- *Duration: Note the length of time that the hot flash or other symptom lasts.*
- *Severity: Score on a scale of 1 to 5, to represent moderate to severe.*

Trigger Tracking:

- *Diet: Foods and beverages taken before symptoms.*
- *Environment: Physical activity, temperature, or stressful situations.*
- *Lifestyle factors include emotional mood, physical activity, and sleep quality.*

Symptom Types:

- *The intensity, frequency, and duration of hot flashes.*
- *Additional symptoms include mood swings, sleep disturbances, and night sweats.*

Relief Measures:

- *What Was Beneficial: Note any measure you take to alleviate the condition, such as applying a cold compress or deep breathing.*

Effectiveness:

- *Score the remedy's level of success.*

Extra Information:

- *Emotional Impact: Note any emotions or ideas connected to every event.*

Additional Observations:

Any patterns seen, including heightened symptoms at particular times of day or during stressful situations.

Making a Hot Flash Diary: A Guide

1. Select Your Format:

- Journal or notebook: An easy-to-transport choice.
- Digital applications: Google Sheets, Excel, and even menopause tracking applications.

2. Establish a Model:

- *Columns or Sections: Make sections for the time, date, symptoms, causes, and ways to feel better.*

3. Be Consistent:

- *Daily Update: Try to note symptoms at the same time each day.*
- *Comprehensive Entries: It will be simpler to identify patterns if you are more detailed.*

Advantages of Maintaining a Symptom Log:

- *Identify Triggers: Determine which meals, pastimes, or stresses make the symptom worse.*
- *Track Progress: Focus on how symptoms change over time and assess how well therapies or lifestyle modifications are working.*
- *Improve Interactions with Providers: Exchange comprehensive, unbiased data to assist physicians in efficiently customizing treatments.*
- *Empower Self-Care: Identifying trends and facilitating proactive management, gives a feeling of control.*

One of the most important tools for managing menopause is a Hot Flash Diary and Symptom Journal. It helps women make educated decisions about their health and treatments by providing insightful information about symptom patterns.

CONCLUSION: Thriving Beyond Menopause: Rediscovering Purpose and Passion

Positive Menopausal Changes: A Rejuvenated Self and a New Era of Self-Empowerment

Menopause is a major life change that is frequently seen negatively because of its mental and physical difficulties. However, it also creates opportunities for empowerment, self-discovery, and personal development. Women should welcome menopause as a time of rejuvenation rather than decline by considering these beneficial changes.

1. Elimination of Cyclical Issues

- *Release from Menstrual Cycles: The elimination of monthly menstruation is one of the most noticeable improvements, as it frees people from the discomfort, uncertainty, and preparation that comes with it. This frequently lessens the mental and physical strain that many women experiences.*
- *Emotional Impact: Many women experience more stable emotional well-being during menopause, free from the hormonal swings associated with periods.*

2. A Priority Change

Self-Focus and Personal Growth:

- *When children have grown or professions have stabilized, menopause frequently coincides with a time of life that promotes self-reflection and self-care. Women usually pursue personal growth, rekindle old interests, or find new ones.*
- *Relationship Reevaluation: This stage promotes relationship reevaluation, which can occasionally result in closer bonds with friends, family, or partners—or the bravery to pursue healthier interactions.*

3. Increased Self-Acceptance and Confidence

- *Body Acceptance: Despite physical changes, many women reports feeling more confident and accepting of who they are. This change frequently results from seeing how resilient their bodies are and appreciating the beauty that goes beyond social norms.*
- *Wisdom and Life Experience: A greater sense of wisdom is frequently brought on by menopause. Women often feel more empowered to express their opinions, establish boundaries, and make experience-based judgments.*

4. Emotional and Mental Clarity

- *Letting Go of Expectations: This phase offers a chance to embrace authenticity and let go of social demands. Many women gain emotional clarity and redefine what satisfaction means to them after being released from the pressures of adolescence.*
- *Strength and Resilience: Overcoming the difficulties of menopause builds resilience. Women frequently come out feeling more capable of managing the challenges of life.*

5. Spiritual Development and Interaction

- *Renewed Purpose: Menopause often serves as a period for people to ponder existential or spiritual issues in an effort to find more significance in their lives. This time can help one feel more connected to the planet and themselves.*
- *Reflection and mindfulness: Practices like writing or meditation frequently gain more significance and foster self-awareness and mental health.*

Embracing the Journey:

Menopause is a potent beginning rather than just an end. Through introspection on the positive changes, women may move through this stage with power, purpose, and rejuvenation, coming out with a more profound and comprehensive awareness of their lives and self.

Sustaining a Positive Attitude Throughout Menopause: Individual Development, Innovation, and Self-Belief

1. Put Wellness and Self-Care First

- *Put Your Health First: Get enough sleep, consume a balanced diet, and exercise frequently. These fundamental behaviors enhance mental clarity, vitality, and mood.*
- *Engage in Mindfulness Practices like yoga, meditation, and deep breathing that can help you feel less stressed and have a more optimistic outlook.*
- *Maintain Hydration: Aim for 8–10 glasses of water daily because dehydration can affect mood and focus.*

2. Develop Your Creativity

- *Try painting, writing, gardening, or crafts as new hobbies. In addition to providing a sense of accomplishment, creative expression may be therapeutic.*
- *Participate in classes or workshops: Take lessons in music, dancing, or painting. This fosters creativity connecting you with like-minded individuals.*

- *Regular Journaling: Maintaining a diary promotes self-awareness by assisting with emotional processing and reflection on personal development.*

3. Establish Reasonable Objectives

- *Short-Term Results: Divide more ambitious objectives into smaller, more doable activities. Celebrate your little victories to boost your self-esteem and drive.*
- *Make a vision board to help you visualize your goals to keep you motivated and focused.*
- *Reflect and Adjust: Evaluate your development regularly. Make necessary adjustments to keep objectives in line with your changing priorities,*

4. Promote Emotional Health

- *Practice Gratitude: Record your daily blessings in a gratitude journal. Your perspective changes when you concentrate on what's going well.*
- *Make Connections with Support Systems: Talk to your loved ones, friends, or support groups. Sharing experiences decreases loneliness and increases emotional resilience.*
- *Counseling or therapy: Consulting a mental health specialist can provide you with the skills to*

deal with emotional challenges and foster personal growth.

5. Develop Self-confidence

- *Affirmations: To strengthen resilience and self-worth, use positive affirmations every day.*
- *Consider Your Accomplishments: Make a list of your prior successes and refer to it whenever you feel self-conscious.*
- *Accept Change: Consider menopause as a period of empowerment and rejuvenation. Turn your attention from what is coming to an end to what is possible.*

6. Strengthen Social Bonds

- *Participate in Communities: Join social circles, book clubs, or menopausal support groups. Sharing experiences fosters understanding and empathy.*
- *Reconnect with Old Friends: It is consoling and joyful to strengthen ties.*
- *Volunteer: Giving back to the community creates a feeling of contentment and purpose.*

7. Make Lifelong Learning an investment

- *Pursue Education: To expand your knowledge or acquire new skills, enroll in seminars or online courses.*
- *Read Extensively: Read up on topics like menopause, creativity, and personal growth. Knowledge promotes self-assurance and self-determination.*
- *Keep Your Mind Open: Adopt a learner's perspective on life. Your viewpoint is widened and life is kept interesting by new experiences.*

8. Have Self-Compassion

- *Don't be critical of yourself; instead, be kind to yourself.*
- *Acknowledge Imperfection: Welcome the process of learning, understanding that progress entails both failures and achievements.*
- *Make Joy Your Top Priority: Schedule time for joyful pursuits like dancing, hiking, or listening to music.*

It's important to take care of your physical well-being, encourage creativity, and make personal development investments to keep a happy attitude throughout menopause. You may turn this time into a potent voyage of self-discovery and confidence by accepting change and concentrating on self-compassion.

Enjoy Your Menopausal Journey!!!